Pelvic Congestion Syndrome
Chronic Pelvic Pain and Pelvic Venous Disorders

Professor Mark S Whiteley

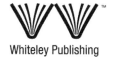

Published by Whiteley Publishing Ltd
First paperback edition 2019
ISBN 978-1-908586-07-0

The information in this book has been supplied by the author and has been published by the publisher in good faith.

Contents

Pelvic Congestion Syndrome - Chronic Pelvic Pain and Pelvic Venous Disorders

Prof Mark S Whiteley

Introduction

In 2000, a patient came to see me in my clinic. She had recurrent varicose veins in her left leg. The patient was the mother of a local family doctor and she had previously had her veins treated in the same leg on two occasions by a very famous varicose veins surgeon in London.

At that time, I had just introduced endovenous surgery (pinhole surgery where veins are burned with heat rather than pulled out by stripping) into the UK. Although I had not proven it at this stage, I already knew that when veins were cut and pulled out, they grew back in most patients - a process called neovascularisation or "strip-tract revascularisation." When this occurs, the new veins do not develop valves and so are instantly new varicose veins all over again. It was another seven years before I published the paper proving this in the British Journal of Surgery.

Therefore, when I examined this patient, I told her that I was certain that her varicose veins had recurred because she had previously had stripping, and her veins had grown back again. I had seen it so many times before it appeared obvious to me.

The patient went next door to see my specialist vascular technologist, Judy Holdstock, who later came to see me with the results of this test. Although called a "vascular technologist" at the time, Judy has spent years specialising in veins with me.

Judy showed me that the stripping had been successful in this patient, with no sign of any regrowth of the stripped veins. However, the recurrent varicose veins on the inner thigh and inner calf were not arising from the usual place in the groin but were coming from veins on the inside of the upper thigh, next to the patient's vulva and vagina.

Not sure why this might be the case, Judy went on to perform a pelvic ultrasound scan. This showed great big varicose veins in the pelvis, with varicose veins emerging through the pelvic floor and out into varicose veins in her labia and upper thigh.

It was this patient who started my interest in pelvic varicose veins. Our research into this fascinating area at The Whiteley Clinic has now been progressing over 20 years.

During this time, we have found that these pelvic varicose veins were almost always caused by pelvic venous reflux (which I will explain later in this book). This pelvic venous disorder, and associated pelvic varicose veins, is a major cause of leg varicose veins in women and some men. We have also found that they cause intimate varicose veins in the vulva and vagina in women (we already knew about varicose veins around the testicles in men!) and that they are associated with haemorrhoids.

Furthermore, we found that pelvic venous reflux can be the source of chronic pelvic pain and other pelvic symptoms that are lumped together under the term "pelvic congestion syndrome", discovering along the way that this is virtually ignored by gynaecologists to the detriment of many of their patients.

We have developed the gold standard technique for finding this pelvic venous reflux and pelvic varicose veins, and for directing treatment. We have also championed treatment that can be performed under local anaesthetic as a walk-in, walk-out procedure, and have set up a dedicated unit for this in our clinic in Bond Street, London.

When I started presenting our research in the early 2000's, there was virtually no interest in this sort of pelvic venous reflux disorder amongst phlebologists and venous surgeons. However, over the last decade, interest has grown exponentially in the venous world, and now every venous meeting has at least one section dedicated to pelvic congestion syndrome and pelvic venous reflux. I have recently been part of the international committee producing the UIP clinical guidelines for the investigation and treatment of pelvic congestion syndrome, and these were published in August 2019.

However, the vast majority of patients who have this problem are still ignored by the system as doctors and nurses in most countries still fail to recognise that pelvic congestion syndrome even exists.

This book is written for patients with pelvic congestion syndrome, whichever one of the manifestations they might have, members of the public who are interested in these medical conditions, and healthcare professionals who want to know more about this fantastically interesting and growing area of medicine.

Chapter 1

Pelvic Congestion Syndrome – is it a real problem?

Many people – even those trained in medicine or nursing – do not really know what "Pelvic Congestion Syndrome" is!

It is shocking to know that research has shown that:

- 1 in 3 (30%) women attending gynaecology outpatients in the UK with chronic pelvic pain have pelvic congestion syndrome. However, virtually none get the correct diagnosis nor treatment. This is mirrored in many other western countries.

- 1 in 6 (16.7%) women with leg varicose veins have them arising from pelvic varicose veins (pelvic congestion). However, virtually none are investigated nor treated by varicose veins surgeons. Hence their leg varicose veins keep coming back again when only the leg varicose veins are treated. This is a major reason why patients often think that "varicose veins always come back".

- Varicose veins of the vulva, labia and vagina are an outward sign of pelvic congestion. However, most gynaecologists, family doctors and midwives tell patients that there is nothing that can be done for these intimate varicose veins. They usually follow up this incorrect information with the equally erroneous advice that they will "get better by themselves" or that the best treatment is to wear supportive pants.

- Haemorrhoids (piles) are often outward signs of pelvic congestion. However, haemorrhoids (piles) are usually treated by bowel surgeons as if they were part of the bowel.

- Varicoceles (varicose veins around the testicle in men) are a male version of pelvic congestion. However, they are traditionally treated by urologists. Moreover, most doctors who lecture on pelvic congestion syndrome usually still teach that pelvic congestion is a condition found in women only!

- Some of the latest research shows that men with erectile dysfunction taking Viagra could be cured by treating pelvic varicose veins: pelvic congestion syndrome in males.

- Patients suffering from pelvic congestion syndrome often suffer from life changing symptoms which can include any of the following:

  - pelvic venous heaviness and aching

  - discomfort on sexual intercourse

  - irritable bowel syndrome

  - irritable bladder

  - low back pain

  - pain in the lower abdomen on one side or the other or both

  - hip pain

Pelvic congestion syndrome can be diagnosed by a specialist but inexpensive ultrasound scan (transvaginal duplex ultrasound using the Holdstock-Harrison Protocol (see later in this book). If pelvic congestion is found to be the cause, a relatively simple local anaesthetic treatment can cure the condition and associated symptoms. However, most patients aren't even being offered this investigation, never mind treatment for the condition.

So why is there such a lack of knowledge and understanding about pelvic congestion? The answer to this comes down to medical and nursing education.

What most doctors and nurses know about venous conditions

If you talk to doctors or nurses and ask about vein problems, they will almost always think that you are talking about varicose veins or deep vein thrombosis (DVT).

When pushed, they will probably be able to tell you that varicose veins in the legs occur because valves fail in the veins. They will probably then tell you this is due to pressure in the abdomen from being fat, pregnant or constipated, all of which have been disproven over the last 20 years!

It is highly unlikely that they will know that leg varicose veins can come from pelvic varicose veins. What is even more upsetting is that most doctors and surgeons who treat varicose veins will not tell you this either, as they either do not know it, or if they do, they may not understand it, despite research showing that this is a major cause of why varicose veins come back after treatment.

One or two who keep up with the research literature may even talk about venous leg ulcers. If they are up-to-date they will point out that most patients with leg ulcers are not treated properly. They will explain that doctors and nurses are still treating leg ulcers with dressings and compression bandages, despite the NICE clinical guidelines and the randomised controlled trials. These have shown that all patients with venous leg ulcers should be referred for venous duplex ultrasonography and endovenous treatment.

It has been proven that this approach would cure venous leg ulcers faster than compression and dressings and reduce the ulcer recurrence rate.

But few nurses or doctors know this, and even fewer act upon it, preferring to refer patients along historical lines to tissue viability or district nurses for dressings and compression.

If you start talking about pelvic congestion syndrome, not only will most doctors and nurses start looking blank or uncomfortable, but even most specialists such as gynaecologists will act the same. Even though these very specialists deal with women presenting with chronic pelvic pain all the time, the vast majority do not recognise, diagnose nor treat pelvic congestion syndrome.

Indeed, at the time this book is being written, pelvic congestion syndrome does not appear in the list of possible causes of pelvic pain on the Royal College of Obstetricians and Gynaecologists website in the UK. In fact, venous causes of pelvic pain aren't even mentioned as a possible cause of pelvic pain, despite it being present in 30% of these patients!

So, what happens to these patients? They either get misdiagnosed, being told they have "endometriosis" or other causes of their pelvic pain, or they get told there is nothing wrong with them.

Most doctors and nurses would be shocked if you start asking if haemorrhoids are a vein problem as they refer such patients to bowel surgeons. As haemorrhoids appear around the anus, it may seem sensible for bowel surgeons to treat them. However, if you had a varicose vein on your knee, would it be sensible for a knee surgeon to treat it? Of course not.

Accurate diagnoses and successful treatments rely on understanding a condition and sending patients to the correct specialist, not by assuming every condition in one anatomical area of the body comes under one specialist in that anatomical area. Once we know the underlying cause of a condition, we can choose the best specialist to investigate and treat it. Increasing amounts of research has shown that haemorrhoids (varicose veins bulging into the anal canal) are part of pelvic varicose veins or pelvic congestion syndrome.

As in all new areas of interest, self-styled "experts" are always happy to stand up and start talking about a new subject, even when they have little background in it nor comprehension about it. At the current time, many doctors who claim to be specialists in pelvic congestion syndrome, are giving talks or writing articles stating that pelvic congestion is solely a problem of women who have had children.

This is complete nonsense. Not only have we treated multiple women with pelvic congestion who have never been pregnant, but also every doctor and nurse learns in their training that boys can get varicose veins around their testicles from valves failing in their "testicular vein". This is called a varicocele.

Women have ovaries rather than testicles. However, apart from the fact the ovary is in the pelvis and the testicle is in the scrotum, the anatomy is the same. For every man who has a varicocele (and there are tens of thousands operated on every year) there is a woman who has a varicocele around her ovary. This is one of the most basic causes of pelvic congestion syndrome. Therefore, men also have the same venous disorders as women, but because it is visible externally in men, it is not recognised as such.

So how can any specialist who truly understands the subject say it is a problem restricted to women who have had children?

Even the most up-to-date specialists are only just starting to hear about the latest research showing the link between pelvic varicose veins in men and erectile dysfunction.

Looking at all these conditions, venous disorders are causing a problem in somewhere around 50-80% of the adult population. The problem is that doctors and nurses are not recognising them because they have not been trained in venous disorders and do not understand them.

Why are venous disorders misunderstood?

Basically, very few doctors and nurses are interested in venous disorders and their associated conditions. Certainly, in the UK, there is no formal training in venous disorders in the current medical school curricula. Recently, a junior doctor came to see me so I could treat her varicose veins. I asked why she had come all the way to see me rather than have one of her local consultants treat her legs. As a medical student, she would have known several teaching hospital consultants and would have been able to approach any of them.

She told me that in her five years of medical school, she was given a single one-hour lecture on varicose veins! The consultant could not be bothered to turn up and teach the session and so had sent their registrar instead. The registrar had apologised to the students, explaining that they knew nothing about varicose veins nor their treatment.

The registrar had loaded the slides that the consultant had given them and then ran through them, reading out the text. All that was shown was the most basic anatomy thought to be associated with leg varicose veins (now years out of date) and treatment by stripping. As this medical student had previously come to one of my courses, she was well aware that this sort of open surgery, performed under general anaesthetic, was both out of date and also leads to high rates of recurrence.

The problem is that there is little, if any interest in venous disorders or the treatment of venous disorders in the public sector. Many people feel that varicose veins are a "cosmetic problem" and therefore should be dealt with in the private sector. Unfortunately, most of the doctors working in the private sector have trained in the public sector and are still working there, moonlighting to the private sector for one or two sessions a week or at weekends. Hence even though the treatment may be private, most of the doctors working there still have little interest or knowledge in the subject.

Fortunately, there are a few of us who have recognised this and have become vein specialists. I have set up The College of Phlebology through which we run courses, write books (such as this one) and have an annual conference for doctors from around the world who want to specialise in venous disorders.

There is a group of specialists from all around the world who regularly meet at conferences, and we share information and teach delegates who only attend one or two such meetings a year. We publish our own research to share our understanding, and peer review each other's research to make sure the science of phlebology (the study of venous disorders) continues to improve so that the patients can benefit.

Having got that off my chest, we can now concentrate on the subject of this book!

Venous disease or venous disorder?

One final point before we launch into the understanding of pelvic congestion syndrome and pelvic venous disorders, is just to note the use of the terms "venous disease" or "venous disorders".

These two terms can be used interchangeably as "disease" can mean any abnormality that impacts on the structure and/or function of the normal body.

However, it is more normal to think of a "disease" as something that is acquired and a "disorder" as something that results from a normal structure failing. It is not a major point and I often use the term "venous disease". However, for consistency, I am going to try to stick to "venous disorder" in this book.

In this book, I am going to concentrate on pelvic congestion syndrome and how that is associated with chronic pelvic pain and pelvic venous disorders.

Chapter 2

Leg Veins and Pelvic Veins - Concepts

Much of my life in medicine has been spent marvelling at how very intelligent doctors and nurses do not question what they have been taught. As healthcare professionals we are taught by our elders and "betters" who, in turn, were taught by their elders and "betters".

Although this system is excellent for passing on experience and knowledge, it stops many doctors and nurses from asking the simple question - "is that correct?"

Why I have always loved medical research is because this is exactly the question that we ask. When new technology becomes available, or new information is published, we set about re-analysing if what we have been taught and what has always been accepted, is actually true. We often find that it is not.

The huge amounts of information that doctors and nurses need to absorb during their training, often prevents them from thinking about simple concepts for themselves.

One of the simplest concepts in pelvic congestion syndrome and leg varicose veins is venous blood flow back to the heart, and what happens when it goes wrong.

To analyse this, let's start off by considering venous blood flow

Arteries take blood from the heart, to tissues around the body, delivering oxygen and nutrients. Veins bring blood back from the tissues, taking the waste products of tissue metabolism to the liver, lungs and kidneys.

Arterial blood flow isn't a problem because the heart pumps arterial blood at a very high pressure. Blood flows from a place of high pressure to a place of low pressure along what is called a "pressure gradient". Therefore, arterial blood has no problem getting to the extremities – the hands, feet and head.

Unfortunately, on the venous side, by the time the blood has been delivered to the tissues and gone through the capillaries, there is very little pressure left in it. Therefore, there is only a very small pressure gradient from the capillaries back to the heart. As such, venous blood can flow back to the heart from all areas of the body when a body is lying flat.

Also, when standing or sitting, venous blood can flow back to the heart from the head, as gravity works positively with the venous pressure gradient, helping the venous blood flow back "downhill" into the heart.

Similarly, venous blood can also flow back to the heart from the hands and arms as these are more or less at the same level as the heart.

The problem of venous flow occurs in veins below the heart. The low-pressure gradient is not enough to force blood back up the veins against gravity in the sitting or standing position. Hence, for venous blood to flow back to the heart from the feet, legs and pelvis, something must be done to overcome gravity.

This is the background to our analysis.

Venous blood flow back to the heart from legs and pelvis

In order to understand the concepts, we are going to use a series of very simple diagrams. The first is shown in Figure 1.

A network of veins starts in the tissues collecting blood from capillaries, and eventually delivers that blood to the heart. To make the argument simple, we can consider this as a single vein from foot to heart (Figure 1). This vein runs from the foot, up the leg, up through the pelvis, up through the abdomen and eventually into the heart in the chest. Of course, this entails the venous blood flowing uphill against gravity and so, when standing, as we have seen above, this cannot happen. There is only enough pressure in the venous blood to get it from the foot to just above the ankles when in the standing position.

Therefore, we need to pump the blood up these veins against gravity (Figure 2). We have a very efficient series of pumps in the foot and leg which all activate in a co-ordinated manner when we move

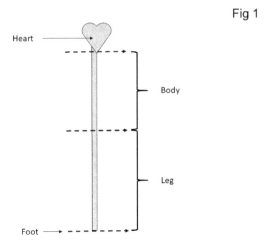

Fig 1

Figure 1: Simple model to understand venous blood flow in the human body. This shows a conceptual single vein running from foot to heart, through the leg and then up through the body.

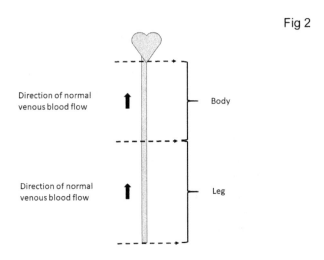

Fig 2

Figure 2: The same simple venous model showing the direction of normal venous blood flow when the muscles in the legs contract, pumping blood upwards against gravity.

and particularly when we walk. There is a pump in the foot, two pumps in the calf and one in the thigh. Some researchers claim that there are more than these four basic leg pumps, but even if there are, the principle is the same.

As we walk, blood is pumped in a coordinated fashion from the foot, up through the leg and into the pelvis. Once in the pelvis, a combination of inertia, blood being pumped from the other leg and respiratory movements complete the pumping process, returning venous blood to the heart.

However, if we stop moving, or when the leg muscles relax between strides, it would be logical to think that blood would fall back down the veins towards the foot with gravity. Therefore, the second essential element of the vein pump are the venous valves. These one-way valves open when blood rushes upwards through the veins, but close as soon as blood starts to fall back down them (Figure 3).

These valves occur every 8-10 cm in the leg veins. They are simple paired flaps of thin tissue, called leaflets, that are attached to the vein wall in a blind ending "sac", very similar to pockets in a coat. They do not actively move by themselves, but they flap open and closed due to the flow of blood around them. When blood flows upwards through the vein, the valves are forced open, pushing the valve leaflets against the vein wall (Figure 3B). When the blood starts to fall back down the veins with gravity, it gets caught by the upper lip of the leaflet, forcing the valve leaflets away from the vein wall and getting caught in the "pockets". The two valve leaflets open, filling with blood-like pockets that are bulging with sweets, and they completely occlude the vein (Figure 3C). This stops any blood falling back down the vein itself. This process is explained fully in my book "Understanding venous reflux: the cause of varicose veins and venous leg ulcers" (ISBN: 978-1-908586-00-1).

As far as this concept is concerned, we only need to consider blood being pumped back from the foot to the heart. All the way up this venous path, other side veins or "tributaries" join these main veins, bringing venous blood from surrounding organs and tissues. These might be muscles or bones in the legs, or organs in the pelvis and abdomen. As most of these have valves in them, blood only flows from tissues or organs into the main veins and then back to the heart.

Fig 3

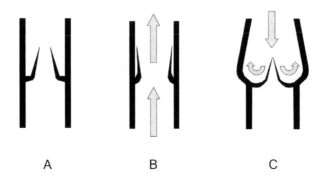

A   B   C

Adapted from: "Understanding Venous Reflux: The Cause of
Varicose Veins and Venous Leg Ulcers " - ISBN: 978-1908586001

Figure 3: Simple diagram of a venous valve and how it works. Each valve has 2 cusps which act like "pockets" attached to the inside of the vein wall. The open part of the pocket is pointing upwards (A). When venous blood is pumped up the leg, the blood pushes the valve leaflets against the vein wall (B). However, when the leg muscles relax, blood falls back down the vein, opening the valve leaflet away from the wall, and effectively closing the valve (C).

However, the problem comes when this system breaks and the venous flow becomes disordered.

The commonest problem that causes the system to break is failure of the valves in the veins. When this happens, blood can fall down the affected vein the wrong way (Figure 4). This is called venous reflux and the vein is said to be "incompetent".

Valve failure and venous reflux

Almost everybody has heard of varicose veins. Varicose veins are a very common condition and, depending on which research you read, affect somewhere between 20 and 40% of the adult population.

Most people know that having varicose veins is something to do with valves failing in the leg veins, although most people cannot picture what this means in real life.

Fig 4

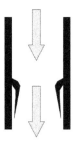

Adapted from: "Understanding Venous Reflux: The Cause of
Varicose Veins and Venous Leg Ulcers " - ISBN: 978-1908586001

Figure 4: Simple diagram of venous valve failure. When a venous valve fails, the leaflets fail to act like pockets, and blood falling down the vein can flow downwards, through the failed valve. Both the valve and this section of vein is said to be "incompetent".

When valves fail in a leg vein, a vein is said to be "incompetent" (Figure 4). This means that blood that has been pumped up an incompetent vein during muscle contraction, falls back down the same vein when the muscles relax. It is the failure of the valves within the vein to stop this backward flow that allows the blood to reflux down the vein towards the foot. The fact that blood is refluxing the wrong way down the vein is what results in the vein being called incompetent.

If the only blood that refluxed down an incompetent vein was the same blood that had just been pumped up it by muscle contraction, it would cause some problems but would not be disastrous.

However, the reason why venous reflux disorder progresses and can cause so much damage, such as inflammation at the ankle and venous ulceration, is that an incompetent vein can also let blood that has already been pumped up into the abdomen and pelvis by other competent veins in the leg, enter and reflux down it (Figure 5). Hence the volume of venous blood refluxing down an incompetent leg vein is far more than the volume of blood that was pumped up it in the first place.

Fig 5

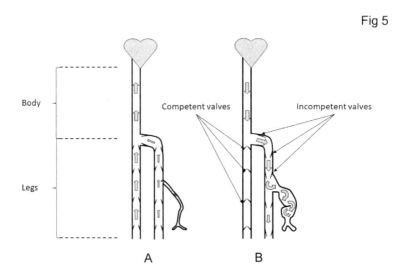

Figure 5: Diagram showing how venous blood flows up the leg veins into pelvic and abdominal veins when the leg muscles contract (A). When the muscles relax, competent valves stop blood falling down competent veins, but incompetent (or "failed") valves let blood reflux down the incompetent vein (B). As there is quite a reservoir of venous blood in the pelvic and abdominal veins that is pumped up from all of the leg veins, there is a large volume of blood that can reflux down the incompetent vein.

When the muscles in the leg contract, pressure increases within the veins of the lower limb and so venous blood flows upwards, through all of the leg veins and into the pelvic veins (Figure 5A). When the muscles relax, blood cannot reflux down competent veins in which the valves have closed, but it can flow down the incompetent vein, because the failed valves allow the blood to reflux with gravity (Figure 5B). Thus, even though the amount of blood going up one vein by itself might not be much, when it becomes incompetent, much greater volumes can end up refluxing down it.

The effects of venous reflux include stretching the vein walls (varicose veins) and inflammation, which can cause pain and damage to tissues below the level of the reflux. As time passes, if the reflux is not stopped, the veins can continue to dilate, allowing increasing amounts of blood to reflux, worsening the symptoms and signs of venous disorder.

This is how venous reflux causes symptoms and signs in patients who have this problem. In leg venous reflux, we often see the results of this incompetence as bulging veins on the surface (varicose veins), swelling of the ankle, venous eczema or red and brown stains around the ankle and, if not treated in time, open sores called venous leg ulcers around the ankles.

This is all pretty well understood by specialists in venous surgery and is why most venous leg ulcers can now be cured by superficial venous surgery. This is the subject of my book "Leg Ulcer Treatment Revolution" (ISBN: 978-1-908586-05-6).

So how does this relate to pelvic congestion syndrome, chronic pelvic pain and pelvic venous disorders?

To understand this, we need to take these same concepts that we have understood in the leg veins and apply them to the next set of veins on the way towards the heart.

Venous reflux in pelvic veins

Most doctors and nurses will be relatively comfortable with the explanations above when related to the leg veins. And yet they do not recognise nor understand pelvic venous reflux. To show how strange this is, we are going to use the simple model derived from the one we looked at earlier.

Venous reflux simple model – leg veins

If we go back to the very basic understanding of a vein running from foot to heart (Figure 1) and blood being pumped from the foot to the heart by muscular contraction (Figure 2), then we just have to imagine the fate of a single blood cell passing along this route.

Let us think of a blood cell starting in the foot. In a competent system such as Figure 2, it will be pumped all of the way to the heart without any problem. However, if the patient has any incompetent veins in the leg, then the blood cell can fall out of the deep system, into the incompetent vein in the superficial venous system, and back down towards the ankle.

Most doctors and nurses will be able to tell you that if venous blood refluxes down incompetent veins arising from the groin or behind the knee, this is called great saphenous vein reflux or small saphenous vein reflux respectively (Figure 6). These are the two most well-known causes of varicose veins and venous reflux disorders of the leg.

Most vascular (that is "arterial") surgeons or other generalists who treat varicose veins, tend to think that these two saphenous veins are the only important veins involved in the development of varicose veins and venous reflux disorders of the lower limb. Hence most of these doctors who are not specialists in venous disorders, perform their own duplex ultrasound scans, and only check and treat these two saphenous veins.

However, those of us who specialise in venous surgery also know that there are some 150 perforating veins in the leg, that take blood from the superficial veins, through the muscle and into the deep veins. They are called "perforating veins" because they perforate the layer of "fascia" (strong connective tissue) that surrounds the muscle.

If the valves in any of these perforating veins fail, then the perforating veins can become incompetent. As they are short and virtually horizontal, there is no pressure gradient to make the venous blood reflux due to gravity. As such, many non-specialist doctors ignore these veins.

However, our research over the years has shown that incompetent perforating veins are a significant cause of varicose veins, venous eczema and venous leg ulcers. It is easy to understand why this is so, using this same simple model.

When the leg muscles contract during walking, pressure in the deep veins increases sharply, in order to pump blood up from the legs to the heart against gravity. The superficial veins under the skin are outside of the muscle, and so there is no change in pressure in these veins during this contraction. Hence, there is a sudden and large pressure gradient from deep veins to superficial veins. Normally the two systems would be separated by the valves in the competent perforating veins. However, if the valves have failed, venous blood can squirt outwards under high pressure through these incompetent perforating veins.

Although the volume of blood squirting outwards through an incompetent perforating vein might be small, the velocity of the jet of blood is high. As energy is more related to the velocity rather than the amount of blood squirting outwards (from school physics: Kinetic energy = ½ mass x velocity^2), the energy of this perforating vein reflux hitting veins and tissue in the lower leg can cause varicose veins and considerable inflammation in the skin and tissue of the lower leg.

So, going back to our consideration of where our blood cell might fall out of our deep veins and reflux out into the superficial veins, and then back towards the foot, we can also add incompetent perforating veins to the saphenous veins in the leg.

Venous reflux simple model – pelvic veins

Because varicose veins are so well-recognised, and the leg is made of bone surrounded by muscle, with subcutaneous fat and skin around it, doctors are quite comfortable with treating veins in the leg. They don't feel that treating these veins is "dangerous" or that there are vital structures that might be damaged during the treatment. As such, even though we do have to teach non-specialist surgeons who want to treat varicose veins properly about incompetent perforating veins, this isn't a great leap for them to learn this new information.

This all changes when we come to pelvic veins.

From a simple conceptual point of view, if you haven't been indoctrinated by medical school and medical training, it is all quite obvious. Going back to our simple model (Figure 6), as our blood cell passes from foot to groin, it can reflux out of the deep veins through any of the incompetent leg veins that we have already discussed. For most doctors who treat varicose veins, that is the end of the story.

However, even a simple understanding of the body shows that they

Fig 6

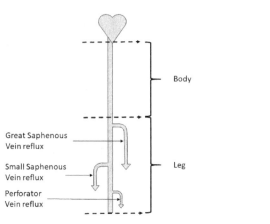

Figure 6: Simple model of superficial venous reflux in the leg. Blood can reflux out of the deep system and into incompetent superficial veins such as the great and small saphenous veins and the perforating veins. These sources of superficial venous reflux are well recognised by most surgeons who treat varicose veins (although many ignore incompetent perforating veins).

are ignoring all of the veins above the groin. As the blood cell flows up from groin to heart, it has to pass up the veins in the pelvis and abdomen. Just as in the leg, there are veins that join the deep system which, if incompetent, can allow our blood cell to reflux out of the deep system and fall downwards because of gravity (Figure 7).

In the lower pelvis, there are the left and right internal iliac veins, and, in the abdomen, there are the left and right gonadal veins. We will look at the actual anatomy of these veins a bit later. The gonadal vein takes blood from the gonad back towards the heart and so in the female it is called the ovarian vein, and in the male it is called the testicular vein.

As you can see from Figure 7, there isn't any real difference between venous reflux in the leg or in the abdomen and pelvis. It is all just blood refluxing out of the deep veins into incompetent peripheral veins. All of these veins should normally be passing blood into the deep vein but the failure of valves allows the reflux.

Fig 7

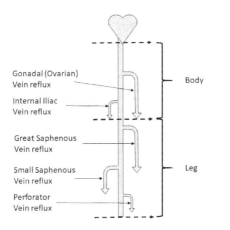

Figure 7: Using the same simple model, it can be seen that there is no conceptual difference between leg vein reflux into incompetent saphenous or perforator veins, and pelvic vein reflux into incompetent gonadal and internal iliac veins. Despite this, the latter are not known about by most doctors who treat varicose veins!

Where doctors and nurses have a problem is that venous reflux inside the body cavity becomes "scary".

There is something quite comforting about considering treatment to veins that are in the leg. The veins are relatively near the surface and if anything goes wrong, it is quite easy to either place compression on the leg or to cut down and operate on the vein directly.

Conversely, veins inside the abdomen and pelvis lie behind the bowel and organs of the abdomen and pelvis. They lie "deep" inside the body and not surprisingly this makes doctors and nurses more anxious about any treatment for them. In addition, unless they are causing an external varicose vein to be seen, such as a varicocele around the male testicle, a varicose vein of the vulva or labia, or a haemorrhoid, then they are not even visible in the normal person. Doctors and nurses find it very difficult to understand and diagnose things that they cannot see.

It is for these reasons that pelvic congestion syndrome has been ignored for so long, and those elements that are known about are assumed to be problems of other systems rather than problems of veins themselves. Hence haemorrhoids are treated by bowel surgeons, varicoceles are treated by urologists and varicose veins of the labia and vulva are largely ignored by midwives and gynaecologists.

Now we have explored the basic concept of why venous reflux in the pelvic veins is very similar to venous reflux in the leg veins, we can look at the anatomy of pelvic veins in more detail. Once we understand the anatomy of the pelvic veins involved in pelvic congestion syndrome, then it will be easier to talk about the symptoms and signs they can cause, how the condition can be investigated and how it can be treated.

Chapter 3

Pelvic Veins - Names and Positions

The term given to the study of the names and positions of structures in the body is called "anatomy". However, many people get put off reading a chapter if you call it "anatomy". It is regarded as rather dry and less interesting than finding out about pelvic congestion syndrome itself.

Unfortunately, it is impossible to discuss pelvic congestion syndrome, to explain the problems it can cause, and how we can treat it, if we don't have a framework showing the position of the different veins that can be involved.

Therefore, this chapter is going to describe the simple layout of pelvic veins in the male and female.

If you do not want to read this in detail at the moment, that is not a problem. Just move on to the next chapter. However, do flip back to this chapter at any time as you go through the rest of the book, just to remind yourself which veins we are talking about.

Pelvic veins in general

The layout of the pelvic veins is very similar in male and female. In fact, the only difference between the two are the veins from the ovaries or testicles. As ovaries and testicles are "gonads" these veins are collectively called the "gonadal veins".

Figure 8 shows the general layout of the veins in the pelvis but does not show the lower end of the gonadal veins. It is only the bottom end of the gonadal veins that varies between males and females. As such this is the general layout in humans without showing the difference between the sexes. We will discuss these differences below.

Although you might think it is easier to describe the veins from the top to the bottom, we will do the reverse. The reason for this is that the normal venous blood flow in living people is up the veins towards

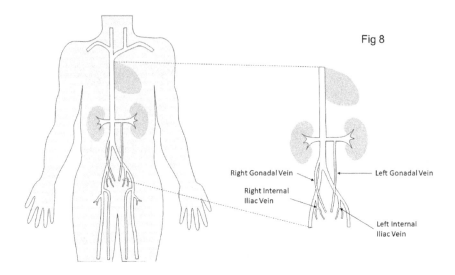

Fig 8

Right Gonadal Vein

Right Internal
Iliac Vein

Left Gonadal Vein

Left Internal
Iliac Vein

Figure 8: Diagram showing the general pattern of the pelvic veins relevant to pelvic congestion syndrome in the human. No detail is shown at the bottom end of the gonadal vein as the general layout is the same in both sexes.

the heart.

We will not go into the different veins in the legs, as we are not looking at vein problems affecting the lower limbs. My other books on varicose veins and leg ulcers go into the leg veins in detail. In this book, we will start at the groin.

On each side, venous blood is pumped out of the leg through a single vein called the common femoral vein (Figure 9). As this leg vein enters the pelvis, it changes its name to the external iliac vein.

The external iliac vein is then joined by a vein emerging from deep inside the pelvis called the internal iliac vein. The internal iliac vein is the final vein collecting venous blood from the pelvic wall, the anus and lower rectum, the bladder, vagina in the female and the prostate in the male.

When the internal and external iliac veins join together on each side, they become the common iliac vein. There is one common iliac vein on each side, the right and left common iliac veins.

These two veins then meet and when they join, they become the inferior vena cava. On the outside, this happens around the level of the belly button (umbilicus).

The inferior vena cava then runs up the back of the abdomen on the front of the spine. It lies next to the aorta which is the major artery in the body.

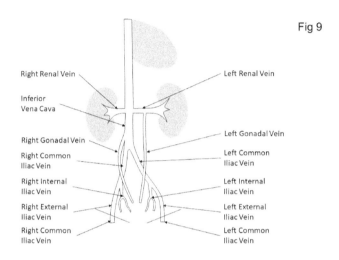

Fig 9

Figure 9: Names of the pelvic veins.

If we forget the gonadal veins for now, the next major veins that are important to understand are the veins from the kidneys. These are called the renal veins. There is one of these on the left and one on the right. The one on the left is longer than the one on the right because the aorta lies between the inferior vena cava and the left kidney. Therefore, the left renal vein runs over the front of the aorta and into the vena cava. This is a very important point and worth remembering for later.

Once the renal veins have joined the inferior vena cava, the inferior vena cava leaves the abdomen, ascending into the chest and heart. This is the end of its course.

The gonadal veins

The gonadal veins are quite different from the general layout of veins in the body. Generally, veins enter into the deep venous system relatively close to the tissue or organ that they are draining. However, in the case of the gonadal veins, the gonads lie low in the pelvis or scrotum, and the veins run up the back of the abdominal wall and then into the deep venous system.

The insertion of these veins into the deep system is asymmetrical. On the right, the gonadal vein enters the inferior vena cava. On the left, the aorta is in the way, and so the left gonadal vein cannot go straight into the inferior vena cava. Instead, it runs up beside the aorta and drains directly into the left renal vein. As noted above, this is a longer vein than the right renal vein as it runs over the front of the aorta. Therefore, the left gonadal vein drains into the renal vein before it passes over the aorta.

If we think about the effect of this on venous blood flow, we can see that venous blood from both left renal vein and left gonadal vein merge, before the left renal vein passes over the aorta. This point is very important in arguments about pelvic congestion syndrome, and what happens if this section of vein gets compressed.

Although the right and left gonadal veins are not symmetrical in their course, this asymmetry is the same pattern in both the male and the female. Both have the left gonadal vein going into the left renal vein and both have the right gonadal vein draining into the inferior vena cava.

It is worthy to note at this early stage that the left gonadal vein is longer than the right gonadal vein. We will see later in this book that the left gonadal vein is more often involved in venous reflux disorder. It is often thought that this is due to the fact that it is significantly longer than the right.

As the left renal vein passes over the front of the aorta, it can be crushed between the aorta and a branch that comes straight out of the aorta called the superior mesenteric artery. This is a rare condition which is called "Nutcracker syndrome". This is one of the rare obstructive conditions that can be associated with pelvic congestion syndrome. We will be discussing these obstructive conditions later in the book.

For now, it is just important to see where these veins enter into the main or deep venous system.

You might wonder why these gonadal veins are so long and meandering compared to other veins in the body. It is well accepted that the reason for this is due to the way that the human develops in the womb.

In the embryo, the gonad is formed very close to the kidney. As the embryo grows into a foetus and then a baby, the gonad moves down the back of the abdomen and into the pelvis. As it does this, it takes the gonadal artery and vein with it. This is essential to keep the blood circulating through the gonad. However, it does mean that both the gonadal artery and vein are very long. In the female, the gonad stays in the pelvis whereas in the male, it should come out of the abdomen and into the scrotum. If it does not, this is called the "undescended testicle".

Now we have gone through the general layout of the pelvic veins, we can move on to look at the small differences in layout between female and male.

Pelvic veins in the female

As you can see in Figure 10, the basic pattern of pelvic veins is present in the female. The only difference is that the ovarian veins start at the ovaries which are within the pelvis and run relatively straight up the back of the abdomen. On the right, the ovarian vein enters the inferior vena cava. On the left, the ovarian vein enters the left renal vein.

Most doctors and nurses who learn this anatomy imagine that this vein is like a "cul-de-sac". Because it entered the pelvis during formation of the foetus, you would think that it would be isolated and not communicate with any of the local pelvic veins.

However, for reasons that are not very well understood, research has shown us that there are many connections between the ovarian vein and other veins in the pelvis. Indeed, there is a very rich network of connecting veins between the lower ovarian veins and many other veins in the pelvis. This network of veins surrounds the pelvic organs such as the rectum, uterus, vagina and bladder as well as the pelvic walls.

The importance of this will become clear later on in this book when we discuss the symptoms and signs of pelvic congestion syndrome and how they can be caused by pelvic varicose veins.

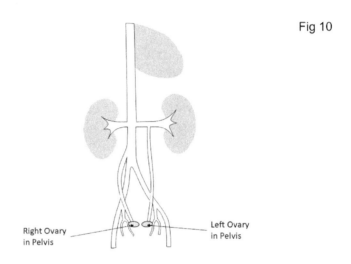

Fig 10

Figure 10: Position of the ovaries in relation to the ovarian (gonadal) veins in the female.

Pelvic veins in the male

Comparing Figure 11 with the previous female pattern of pelvic veins (Figure 10), the differences between the two sexes can be seen. Whereas the ovaries come to rest in the pelvis next to the uterus, in the male, the testicles continue to descend right out of the pelvis. There is a passageway that goes through the muscle at the bottom of the abdominal wall called the "inguinal canal". Provided the testicle descends normally, as a foetus and in the new-born, the testicle passes down through the pelvis, out through the abdominal wall in the inguinal canal and comes to rest in a sac called the scrotum.

As with the ovary, the gonadal artery and vein follow the gonad. In the male these are called the testicular artery and vein.

Once again, you would think that the testicular vein would be a long vein with no attachments in the pelvis. However, research published from The Whiteley Clinic has proven this not to be the case. We have proven that if testicular veins lose their valves and become varicose veins, this can lead to varicose veins in the male pelvis and even varicose veins in the legs. This has revolutionised our understanding of leg varicose veins as well as our understanding of pelvic congestion syndrome.

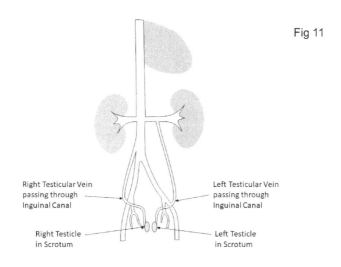

Fig 11

Right Testicular Vein
passing through
Inguinal Canal

Left Testicular Vein
passing through
Inguinal Canal

Right Testicle
in Scrotum

Left Testicle
in Scrotum

Figure 11: Position of the testicles in relation to the testicular (gonadal) veins in the male.

Right jugular vein and right common femoral vein

The description of the pelvic veins above is enough to understand a lot of the discussion and explanation in later chapters about pelvic congestion syndrome and how it causes the signs and symptoms that are associated with it. However, it is also worth pointing out the anatomy of the right internal jugular vein (marked as the "right jugular vein") and right common femoral artery (Figure 12).

These are the two commonest points where the deep venous system can be accessed to treat pelvic congestion syndrome and pelvic varicose veins. Therefore, it is worth having a working knowledge of these two points at this stage. Once again, you can refer back to this chapter later on to refresh your memory if needed.

Now that we have a basic understanding of the anatomy of the pelvic veins, we can start to think about their function in normal people, what can go wrong and what the consequences of that might be. This is the subject of the next chapter.

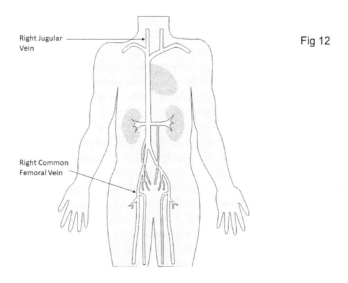

Right Jugular Vein

Fig 12

Right Common Femoral Vein

Figure 12: Figure showing the relative positions of the right jugular vein and right common femoral vein. We will need to know where these 2 veins are when we talk about treatment later.

Chapter 4

Pelvic Vein Function and What Goes Wrong – Reflux, Obstruction and Stasis

Now we have seen the general layout of the pelvic veins in chapter 3, we can start thinking of how the venous blood flows normally and what can go wrong.

There are a great many veins in the abdomen and so we are only going to consider those that are relevant to the understanding of pelvic congestion. We are going to ignore the veins around the bowel, which return through the liver via a special venous system called the "portal venous system".

We are going to concentrate on the veins that we have already looked at in the last chapter.

However, we are going to split the veins up into different groups to help understand the different forces that cause venous blood to return to the heart.

Renal veins (veins from the kidneys)

There are two kidneys, right and left. Kidneys filter the blood, removing excess water as well as a great many other waste products including urea and some other metabolites, and even some drugs. The resulting waste product is urine.

Because the kidneys must filter the blood efficiently, they have a very high blood flow. In fact, physiology experiments have shown that approximately 25% (one quarter) of the whole cardiac output goes to the kidneys. This huge amount of arterial blood flows to the kidneys through the renal arteries.

This high-pressure arterial blood flows through the tissue of the kidneys, where water and metabolites get filtered out of it. As the blood emerges, freshly filtered, from the kidneys, it is collected in small veins that coalesce into the renal vein on each side.

Not surprisingly, the renal veins also have a huge blood flow. Although the pressure is low, being the venous system, virtually the same amount of blood is leaving the kidneys every minute as has arrived in the arteries. The only difference is the bit that has been filtered out to make urine. Therefore, the venous blood flow in the renal veins is both high volume and constant, and it pushes towards the inferior vena cava, and then back to the heart (Figure 13).

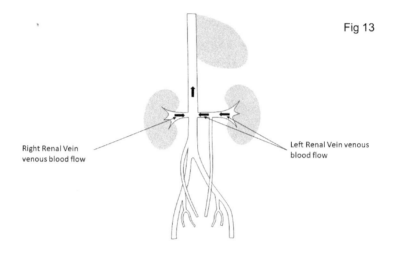

Fig 13

Right Renal Vein venous blood flow

Left Renal Vein venous blood flow

Figure 13: Venous blood flow from the kidneys in the renal veins, is low pressure but very high volume.

Venous flow from the leg veins through the pelvic veins to the heart

Now we are starting to move into a slightly more complex area, and we must understand the dynamics of blood flow during walking, and also when lying flat.

Firstly, we will consider walking. As we discussed in chapter 2, venous blood is pumped up the veins in the legs by muscle action, and then on into the pelvic veins. Blood in the pelvic veins then flows upwards to the heart. Of course, this flow is still against gravity and so there must be a reason that blood flows uphill.

In fact, there is not only one reason. There are several forces in action at the same time.

Imagine what happens in the leg veins when a person is walking. The muscles of the leg contract, squeezing the deep veins. This generates considerable pressure in the venous blood within these veins, so that the blood shoots up the deep veins in the leg. These veins connect through the common femoral vein into the pelvic veins via the external iliac vein (Figure 14).

As venous blood leaves the common femoral vein in the leg and enters the external iliac vein in the pelvis, it has momentum. In addition, it is being pushed by more blood behind it which is also leaving the leg under pressure from the muscle contraction. This is much the same idea as seeing water shooting out of a fountain.

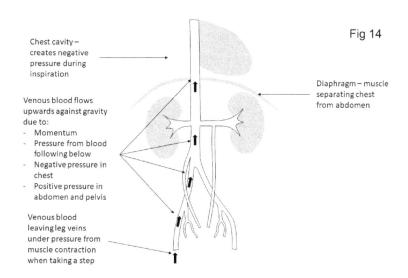

Chest cavity – creates negative pressure during inspiration

Diaphragm – muscle separating chest from abdomen

Venous blood flows upwards against gravity due to:
- Momentum
- Pressure from blood following below
- Negative pressure in chest
- Positive pressure in abdomen and pelvis

Venous blood leaving leg veins under pressure from muscle contraction when taking a step

Fig 14

Figure 14: Diagram showing the forces on the venous blood entering the pelvic veins, enabling it to flow uphill against gravity and so into the heart.

This upward flow against gravity is assisted by the action of breathing. When we breathe in, there is negative pressure in the chest. Blood in the pelvis is at normal atmospheric pressure (+ any pressure remaining from the muscle contraction in the leg) and the negative pressure helps create a pressure gradient for venous blood to flow upwards against gravity. This is supplemented by any increase in intra-abdominal pressure during respiration or other activities such as straining (for example when lifting a heavy weight or when constipated).

When the leg muscles relax and the jet of blood from the leg stops, there is a jet of blood coming from the other leg, from the muscle contraction on that side (Figure 15). This change over happens every step that we take. I often imagine this to be like 2 pistons working alternately to make sure a constant flow continues up the central inferior vena cava and back to the heart.

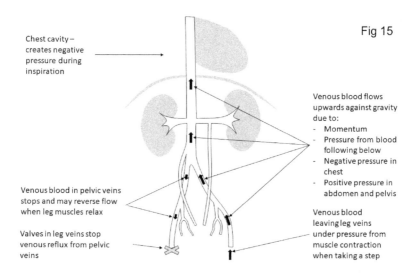

Chest cavity – creates negative pressure during inspiration

Fig 15

Venous blood flows upwards against gravity due to:
- Momentum
- Pressure from blood following below
- Negative pressure in chest
- Positive pressure in abdomen and pelvis

Venous blood in pelvic veins stops and may reverse flow when leg muscles relax

Valves in leg veins stop venous reflux from pelvic veins

Venous blood leaving leg veins under pressure from muscle contraction when taking a step

Figure 15: Diagram showing that when the leg relaxes and blood starts to reflux in the pelvic veins, contraction of muscles in the other leg replaces the upward flow in the inferior vena cava.

Finally, when we lie down gravity does not play a part, and blood flows the right way through these veins. The reason for this is that there is no gravity to overcome, and so blood emerging from all of the tissues in the legs, pelvis and abdomen is at higher pressure than the pressure in the chest. Hence venous blood flows from the tissues and back to the heart.

Venous flow in the gonadal veins

In the normal person, venous blood flows up the gonadal veins (Figure 16). The veins are relatively small compared to the renal veins or inferior vena cava, as the blood flow to the gonads is not particularly high and so there is not a huge volume of venous blood to be removed each minute.

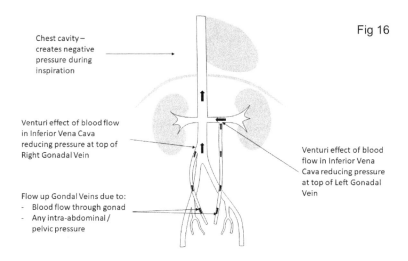

Fig 16

Chest cavity – creates negative pressure during inspiration

Venturi effect of blood flow in Inferior Vena Cava reducing pressure at top of Right Gonadal Vein

Venturi effect of blood flow in Inferior Vena Cava reducing pressure at top of Left Gonadal Vein

Flow up Gondal Veins due to:
- Blood flow through gonad
- Any intra-abdominal / pelvic pressure

Figure 16: Diagram showing the forces on venous blood in the gonadal veins, forcing it to flow uphill against gravity, and back to the heart.

Venous blood emerging from the gonad tissue has a residual pressure, and this is the first element of pressure pushing blood up the gonadal vein. Any intra-abdominal or intra-pelvic pressure from breathing, or other movements such as straining, will also add to this pressure. Negative pressure in the chest during breathing increases the pressure gradient from gonad to heart, further helping the flow up the gonadal veins.

Finally, although each of the gonadal veins has a different insertion into the main venous system, they both have a junction with a high flow, large volume vein which has constant forward flow towards the heart (Figure 16).

On the right, the gonadal vein empties into the inferior vena cava. As explained above, due to the alternating "piston-like" pumping of venous blood from the legs when walking, the upward flow in the inferior vena cava is fairly constant. The fast flow in the inferior vena cava creates a low-pressure area at the junction of the right gonadal vein, by the Venturi effect. The Venturi effect is a reduction of pressure outwards when a fluid is flowing fast. Because of the fast-flowing nature of blood in the inferior vena cava, this creates an increased pressure gradient between the right ovarian vein and the inferior vena cava, helping venous blood to flow up the gonadal vein against gravity.

On the left, the gonadal vein empties into the left renal vein. As described above, the left renal vein has a very high flow because of the enormous blood supply to the kidney. As such, all the same forces are at work in the left gonadal vein including the Venturi effect at its junction with the left renal vein.

Venous flow in the internal iliac veins

The internal iliac veins are quite short. They are made by a great many tributaries arising from many areas in the lower pelvis. Some of these veins come from the muscles in the pelvic wall. Some come from the lower rectum and anus. Some from the vagina and bladder. Some also communicate with veins from outside of the pelvis including leg veins, perineal veins and veins of the external genitalia. In the male, they also drain the prostate and penis.

As such, the forces that cause upward flow in these veins are many and varied. They include the residual pressure in the venous blood as it emerges from the organs and tissues that are drained by the tributaries that join to form the internal iliac vein. The veins that communicate with the legs transmit the pulses of high-pressure venous flow when the muscles of the legs contract during walking. The same is found in tributaries draining the buttock and pelvic muscles, as these muscles also pump venous blood at high pressure when they contract during movement.

Any raised pressure in the pelvis from breathing or movement, coupled with reduced pressure in the chest during inspiration, also helps the pressure gradient in these veins and hence helps flow upwards towards the chest.

There may also be an element of Venturi effect when the internal iliac veins join the external iliac veins to form the common iliac vein on each side. The fast flow of the venous blood in the external iliac vein passing over the open end of the internal iliac vein can cause a reduction in pressure, aiding a pressure gradient for blood to flow upwards.

So now we can understand the general flow of blood in the pelvic veins in normal people. So, what can go wrong?

Valves in the pelvic veins

As can be seen from the explanations above, the flow of venous blood in the veins in the legs follow much more simple principles than the flow of venous blood in the pelvic veins. Having said this, although the principles are simple, the very high recurrence rates that most patients experience when treated by non-specialist doctors shows that even the simpler leg veins are not well understood by many doctors!

In the legs, all the significant veins have valves. In veins, venous valves are very simple. We have already briefly touched on this previously. The valves are arranged in pairs of leaflets which are a bit like pockets in a coat. As we have seen, when blood is pumped upwards by movement, the valves open passively (Figure 3). Conversely, when blood starts to fall back down the vein, the flow catches the edge of the valve leaflets, causing it to close (Figure 3). This is a passive process with the valve leaflets fluttering open and closed purely by the direction of the flow of blood.

For many reasons, often associated with familial factors, these venous valves can fail (Figure 4). When this happens, blood starts to flow the wrong way through the vein either due to gravity (passive or "diastolic" reflux) or during the muscle contraction of the leg (active or "systolic" reflux). Although leg veins can exhibit both sorts of reflux, when pelvic veins are incompetent, they mainly show a passive reflux due to gravity. Therefore, in this book on pelvic congestion, we can forget about active ("systolic") venous reflux.

In legs, when veins become incompetent and venous blood refluxes the wrong way down them, several symptoms or signs can develop. Initially, there may be nothing to notice. However, with time, as the condition deteriorates, either the venous reflux starts dilating veins near the surface (varicose veins) or it impacts on the tissues lower down the leg causing inflammation. This inflammation can cause tired or aching legs, thread veins, venous eczema, red or brown stains around the ankles and even leg ulcers. If there are no visible bulging veins on the surface, this can be called "hidden varicose veins", a term I introduced in 2011 in a previous book.

So how does this relate to the pelvic veins?

You would think that the basic layout would be the same. You would think that all the veins in the pelvis would similarly have valves in them. Unfortunately, this is not the case.

The external iliac veins, common iliac veins and inferior vena cava do not usually have valves. It may be that the huge flow of blood being pumped out of the legs, augmented by breathing, means that valves are unnecessary. Whatever the reason, it is uncommon to have a valve in any of these veins. Despite this, these veins do not reflux in the same way that leg varicose veins do.

The major reason for this lack of reflux is that in the normal person, the valves in the veins at the top of the leg stop any reflux from these major pelvic veins into the leg veins. Of course, when these valves fail at the top of the legs, blood from the major pelvic veins falls into the legs, which can result in the development of the symptoms and signs listed above. If this subject is of interest to you, then you will find a more detailed explanation in the book "Understanding Venous Reflux: The cause of varicose veins and venous leg ulcers".

So now let's look at the other veins in the pelvis and abdomen

The renal veins, from the kidneys, similarly do not have valves. This is because they are essentially a "cul-de-sac". The kidneys have a huge blood supply from the renal arteries. The arterial blood goes through the kidney tissue and comes out of the kidneys into the renal veins.

There is a very healthy one-way flow along the renal veins and into the inferior vena cava. Hence there is no need for a valve here.

This then only leaves the gonadal veins and the internal iliac veins to discuss. These are the two sets of veins that are important in pelvic congestion syndrome.

Valves in the gonadal veins

As we saw in chapter 3, the gonadal veins are long veins that run up the back of the abdominal wall. The left gonadal vein is longer than the right gonadal vein. Because these veins are long and have much lower flow rates than the major pelvic and abdominal veins we have discussed above, they do have valves. A normal gonadal vein has a series of valves usually spaced some 5-10 cm apart.

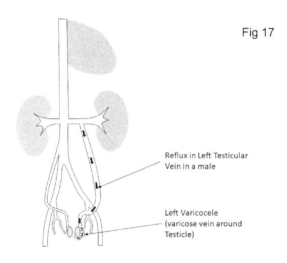

Fig 17

Reflux in Left Testicular Vein in a male

Left Varicocele (varicose vein around Testicle)

Figure 17: Diagram showing how reflux in an incompetent testicular vein causes a testicular varicocele.

Just as in the venous valves in leg veins, these valves open and close depending on the blood flow across them. This make sure that blood only goes up and does not fall down the vein.

If the valves do fail, then the gonadal vein can become incompetent and blood can reflux down the gonadal vein.

In the male, this reflux in the testicular vein causes a varicose vein around the testicle called a varicocele (Figure 17).

In the female, this reflux in the ovarian vein causes a similar "varicocele" or varicose vein around the ovary (Figure 18). However, unlike in the male where the testicle is distant from the rest of the pelvic organs and veins, the ovary is in the middle of the pelvis and the ovarian vein has lots of other veins connecting to it. Therefore, this ovarian varicocele can cause varicose veins to develop on structures around it. Depending on which veins dilate, this can affect the bowel, vagina, bladder, pelvic wall, pelvic floor or even out to the labia, anal canal and legs.

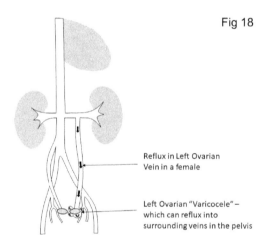

Fig 18

Reflux in Left Ovarian Vein in a female

Left Ovarian "Varicocele" – which can reflux into surrounding veins in the pelvis

Figure 18: Diagram showing how reflux in an incompetent ovarian vein causes an ovarian varicocele. Unlike in the male, the ovarian varicocele is connected to many veins in the pelvis and so this reflux can spread widely into other veins in the pelvis.

You will already be able to see the distribution of which structures can be affected by pelvic congestion syndrome, even when it is due to an ovarian varicocele – the simplest form of this condition. In addition, by understanding that venous reflux is the underlying problem, you'll be able to start to understand how the symptoms and signs of pelvic congestion syndrome occur.

Very importantly, you will also start to understand that whereas a varicocele is obvious in the male because it is outside and visible, the "female varicocele" around the ovary is deep inside the pelvis and therefore cannot be seen with the naked eye. This is a major reason as to why it has been ignored for so long by doctors and nurses.

However, back to the underlying cause. So why do these valves in the gonadal veins fail?

Just as in the leg varicose veins, we really don't know. However, there is certainly a very big familial component as these vein disorders run in families. Many doctors think that these valves fail because of an obstruction or compression higher up the vein. We will be discussing this in detail later. Although this can happen, our research at The Whiteley Clinic has shown that in reality, obstruction and compression is rarely the cause of the reflux. Not only have we shown that some of the tests that are commonly used by doctors can give the wrong results, but we have also recently shown that the valves start failing from the bottom of the ovarian vein and not from the top.

This mirrors the research we published in 2001 showing the same pattern in the leg veins, during the development of varicose veins. Although leg varicose veins have always been thought to be a problem with pressure in the pelvis (usually put down to pregnancy, constipation, heavy-lifting or pelvic tumours), such an obstruction of venous flow from the legs would result in the top valve in the leg veins giving way first. The pressure would then pass on to the next valve down, which would then fail and so on. This progression of varicose veins is called descending reflux, as the valves fail like dominoes one after another.

In reality this almost never happens. In fact, venous reflux progresses in exactly the opposite way. We have proven that the first valve to give way is usually lower in the leg. This has some effect either by altered flow or by dilation of the vein, which affects the next valve higher up. When this fails, the same process is then transferred to the next valve higher and the reflux progresses in an ascending pattern.

Although this is much less logical, careful studies with duplex ultrasonography have shown it to be correct. Once again this is more fully discussed in my book "Understanding Venous Reflux: The cause of varicose veins and venous leg ulcers".

We have presented research from The Whiteley Clinic at international meetings showing that the same ascending pattern is found in ovarian veins. In fact, a descending pattern is rarely found. This shows that in most patients with ovarian vein reflux at least, compression of the vein at the top causing reflux to occur below (the so called "nutcracker syndrome" - see below) is rarely the cause.

This is very worrying as there is a group of doctors involved in pelvic congestion syndrome treatments who believe that compression syndromes are far more common than we have found them to be, and who recommend stents to open the "compressed" veins in these patients. This is probably incorrect in many, if not the majority, of patients, leading not only to wasted expense but potentially to long-term complications that are unnecessary. We will return to this to discuss it more fully later in this book.

For those who are uncertain as to which is more likely, an ascending pattern due to familial propensity to valve failure, or a descending pattern of valve failure due to obstruction and vein compression at the top of the vein, there is a further simple argument that supports our view.

For decades now, the male version of the incompetent gonadal vein is a varicocele around one or both testicles. This can ache, often worries males who have it but more importantly, the heat from the blood in the varicocele can reduce fertility by abnormally heating the testicle. Therefore, a varicocele needs treatment.

The usual treatment for a varicocele is an operation to tie the testicular vein and stop the reflux. This has been done by urologists for decades and rarely causes problems. More recently this has been done by interventional radiologists who block the vein from the inside using embolic coils (we will be discussing this at length later in the book).

If the reflux in the testicular vein in these males was due to obstruction of the vein higher up due to compression syndromes, then these men would get worse with this operation rather than better. We know from many years of experience that this is not the case and so we know that such compression syndromes are actually very rare.

As this condition mirrors the female ovarian varicocele and associated pelvic congestion syndrome, it is highly likely to be the same in females with ovarian varicoceles secondary to ovarian vein reflux.

We will return to this later.

Valves in the internal iliac veins

The presence or absence of valves in the internal iliac veins and tributaries forming the internal iliac veins is quite controversial. Some authorities say there are no valves in these veins, others that they do contain valves.

As we will see later, the gold standard test for these veins is a transvaginal duplex ultrasound scan, using the Holdstock-Harrison protocol. This specialist ultrasound scan can show the blood flowing in veins, including which direction the blood is flowing. Using this test, venous reflux can be seen if present, and so competent internal iliac veins can be distinguished easily from incompetent ones. The incompetent iliac veins show huge amounts of venous reflux on a transvaginal venous duplex ultrasound scan, provided the Holdstock-Harrison protocol is used.

It doesn't really matter if there are valves or not in these veins, provided the internal iliac vein is competent. Whatever the mechanism, if the vein becomes incompetent and exhibits gross reflux, symptoms and signs often occur downstream. The symptoms and signs then usually get better when the vein is treated and the reflux stopped, showing a good correlation between the incompetent vein and the clinical problem.

Therefore, all that is important is whether the vein is competent or not. Whether this competence is due to functioning venous valves, or there is a one-way mechanism for venous flow that has not been described yet, is not relevant. In reality, functioning valves that fail is the most likely explanation for why internal iliac veins might be competent or incompetent.

Venous reflux as a cause of pelvic congestion syndrome

So, what we have seen from this chapter so far is that pelvic venous reflux is really a problem of one or more of the four veins, right or left gonadal veins and right or left internal iliac veins.

Of course, we must remember that veins are draining blood from organs and tissues, and so when we talk about these major veins, we have to remember they are made up from many much smaller veins that join together. These smaller veins or tributaries arise from organs and tissues in the area, drained by the whole system feeding into each of these major veins.

So, when any of these major veins become incompetent and venous blood refluxes down them, the venous reflux can pass into multiple different channels, depending which set of valves has failed. For instance, if the valves in the veins draining from the vulva into the internal iliac vein have failed, venous reflux will result in varicose veins of the vulva. Conversely, if valves fail in the veins draining from the anus into the internal iliac vein, venous reflux will result in haemorrhoids (piles).

In addition, it is important to remember that just as varicose veins in the legs can have many different patterns, pelvic vein reflux can also have many different patterns.

Published research from The Whiteley Clinic has shown the commonest pattern of reflux is reflux in the left ovarian vein and both internal iliac veins in women (Figure 19). This is probably the same in men but because many men have varicoceles treated in early life, and because transvaginal venous duplex ultrasound scan is obviously not possible in men, it is more difficult to know for sure.

A recent research paper from an excellent unit in Turkey has shown that male patients who have varicoceles are more likely to have haemorrhoids, and vice versa. Therefore, there is a clear link between the two conditions.

It is without doubt that venous reflux in these pelvic veins is the major cause of pelvic congestion syndrome in most patients. However, apart from venous reflux, there are two other elements of venous disease that we must discuss at this stage. These are venous obstruction and venous stasis. For those readers who are interested in venous disorders, and more specifically how venous reflux, obstruction and stasis, specifically in the legs, can cause the patient symptoms and signs, these are also discussed in detail in my book "Leg Ulcer Treatment Revolution".

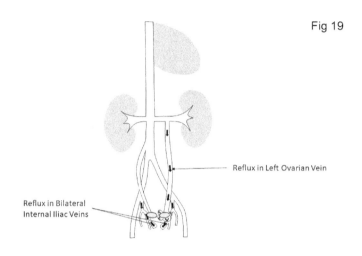

Fig 19

Reflux in Left Ovarian Vein

Reflux in Bilateral
Internal Iliac Veins

Figure 19: Diagram showing the commonest pattern of pelvic venous reflux – reflux in the left ovarian vein and bilateral internal iliac veins.

Venous obstruction and compression as a cause of pelvic congestion syndrome

Many doctors are fixated on the idea that pelvic congestion syndrome is caused by venous obstruction in a large proportion of patients.

What we mean by "venous obstruction" is a narrowing or blockage of a vein higher up towards the heart that increases the resistance to venous blood flow. This makes it harder for the venous blood to flow through the affected vein. These doctors then think that the increased resistance causes the venous blood to find another way back to the heart. If these alternative routes mean that blood has to flow the wrong way down one or more veins to get to where it needs to go, then it can only do so by bursting through the valves and making the alternative

55

vein incompetent.

A lot of doctors find such thoughts quite attractive, as they like to have a logical reason as to why valves fail. Extra venous pressure on the valve sounds like an excellent reason why it might fail.

Of course, we have already seen that this is not the case in leg varicose veins (see above) as most leg varicose veins are caused by primary failure of the valves lower down in the leg. Similarly, recent prize-winning research from The Whiteley Clinic has shown that most patients with pelvic congestion syndrome have also got primary valve failure without any other obstructive or compressive cause.

Although obstruction from compression is a very uncommon cause for the symptoms and signs of pelvic congestion syndrome, they can exist in uncommon cases. Therefore, I will explain each of them here to help discussion later in the book.

Nutcracker syndrome (NCS)

As we saw in chapter 3, the inferior vena cava is separated from the left kidney by the aorta (Figure 20). Therefore, the left renal vein has to travel from the left kidney over the aorta before it drains into the inferior vena cava. The left gonadal vein drains into the renal vein, on the kidney side of the aorta. As the renal vein passes over the aorta, a major branch of the aorta called the superior mesenteric artery (a major blood supply to the gut) passes in front of the renal vein (Figure 20).

At the point where the left renal vein passes over the aorta, but under the superior mesenteric artery, a narrowing of this angle can squash the renal vein and compress it (Figure 21). This is likened to a "nutcracker". When this happens, the pressure in the left renal vein will increase due to the blood flow in being obstructed as it passes over the aorta. The only escape for the blood will be down the left gonadal vein.

In this situation, it is often thought that the pressure bursts through the valve at the top of the left gonadal vein, followed then by the other valves lower down. This would allow the venous blood to escape from the left renal vein and back up through the other veins in the pelvis. This incompetence would progress as a descending pattern of reflux (top valve failing first).

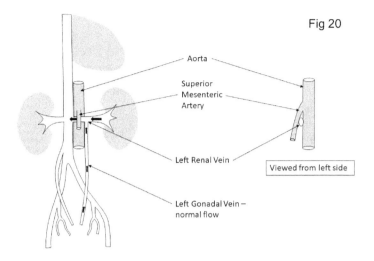

Fig 20

Aorta

Superior
Mesenteric
Artery

Left Renal Vein

Viewed from left side

Left Gonadal Vein –
normal flow

Figure 20: Diagram showing the left renal vein passing over the aorta and under the superior mesenteric artery before joining the inferior vena cava.

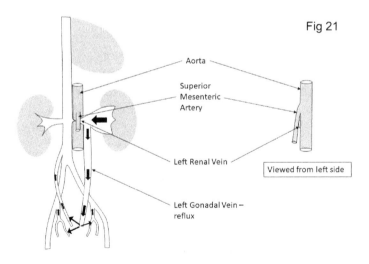

Fig 21

Aorta

Superior
Mesenteric
Artery

Left Renal Vein

Viewed from left side

Left Gonadal Vein –
reflux

Figure 21: Diagram showing nutcracker syndrome. Compression of the left renal vein between aorta and superior mesenteric artery creates resistance to flow and increases pressure in the left renal vein. It escapes by bursting through valves in the left gonadal vein and refluxing down into the pelvis, to find other routes back to the heart.

When this happens, high volumes of venous blood from the left kidney and left renal vein rush down the left gonadal vein. In the female, this refluxing flow in the left ovarian vein dilates veins in the pelvis causing pelvic congestion syndrome, as blood flows into the network of pelvic veins to find a route up the right ovarian vein or either internal iliac vein.

In the male, blood rushing down the left testicular vein will cause a varicocele and similarly will open the network of veins in the left inguinal canal and pelvis, so blood can find a way out of this high-flow network.

As noted earlier, the kidneys have a very high blood supply. Therefore, if the left renal vein is obstructed by the compression of the superior mesenteric artery in a true nutcracker syndrome, the back pressure in the left renal vein will raise pressure in the left kidney capillaries, causing pain in the left flank and back. In addition, the high pressure of blood in the capillaries in the kidney itself causes blood to pass into the urine. The amounts are usually microscopic and so a test on the urine is needed rather than just looking for blood with the naked eye.

In normal practice, our research at The Whiteley Clinic has shown that nutcracker syndrome is often mis-diagnosed by doctors still using magnetic resonance imaging (MRI), magnetic resonance venography (MRV), computerised tomography (CT scanning) or venograms. When we use the transvaginal venous duplex ultrasound scan (the Holdstock-Harrison protocol) with extended abdominal views (the Holdstock-White protocol) we have shown that the diagnosis using these other tests is often incorrect.

As we will discuss later, our prize-winning research has shown that the appearance of nutcracker syndrome on these other tests is usually caused by blood refluxing down an incompetent left gonadal vein. This diversion of blood falling down an incompetent vein causes the left renal vein to collapse and appear to be narrowed. If the patient is tipped head down to counter the gonadal vein reflux, the "compressed" renal vein opens up again, and the appearance of nutcracker syndrome disappears.

We have named this "pseudo-nutcracker" rather than nutcracker. Pseudo-nutcracker also explains the discrepancy between the large proportion of women being diagnosed with nutcracker syndrome in some units, versus the very few patients who have problems when left gonadal vein reflux is treated successfully both in females, for pelvic congestion syndrome, and in males, with left testicular varicocele. In a true nutcracker syndrome, blocking the left gonadal vein to stop the reflux would prevent blood escaping the left kidney, and so the patient would be in agony as soon as the procedure was performed.

Therefore, the diagnosis of nutcracker syndrome should only be made in special circumstances. The patient has to be shown to have severe pain in the left flank and back, and the renal vein appear compressed even when the patient is tipped head down during examination. As most MRI and CT machines do not allow for tipping the patient, you can already see that using these tests to look for pelvic congestion syndrome is sub-optimal.

May-Thurner syndrome (MTS)

The second major venous obstruction or compression in pelvic veins is called the May-Thurner syndrome (Figure 22). As in the nutcracker syndrome, May-Thurner syndrome is a consequence of the veins lying to the right side of the aorta, and both blood vessels lying on the spine. When the aorta splits into two arteries called the common iliac arteries, the right common iliac artery has to pass over the left common iliac vein to get to the right leg (Figure 22).

Although in most people this is not a problem, in some people, the artery flattens the vein against the bone of the spine. Once again, this compression can cause a resistance to blood flow up the vein. In May-Thurner syndrome, if the narrowing is enough to raise the pressure in the veins, the venous blood must escape down the left internal iliac vein, run across veins in the pelvis and then usually up the right internal iliac vein. This causes a dilation of veins in the pelvis, giving the appearance of pelvic congestion syndrome.

Once again, research has shown that most people with reflux in the left internal iliac vein have primary valve reflux and there is no increased resistance from a true May-Thurner obstruction.

However, a true May-Thurner syndrome can occur and, in such cases, the most serious outcome is not pelvic congestion syndrome but is a blood clot forming at this point. A blood clot in the vein is called a deep vein thrombosis (DVT). When a DVT forms in the left common iliac vein, it is very serious. The common iliac vein is a large and major vein and so the clot would be very large. Also, it would stop the outflow of blood from the left leg and would cause considerable swelling and pain of that leg.

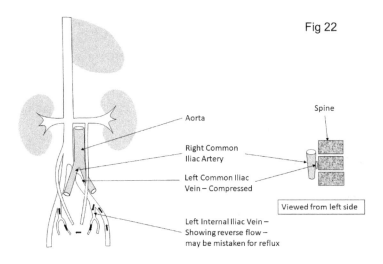

Fig 22

Aorta

Right Common
Iliac Artery

Left Common Iliac
Vein – Compressed

Spine

Viewed from left side

Left Internal Iliac Vein –
Showing reverse flow –
may be mistaken for reflux

Figure 22: Diagram showing May-Thurner syndrome. The right common iliac artery passes over the left common iliac vein. If it compresses the vein against the spine enough to cause a resistance to venous flow, venous blood has to escape down the left internal iliac vein. However, the commonest cause of reflux in the left internal iliac vein is primary reflux without any compression.

Fortunately, just as with nutcracker syndrome, May-Thurner syndrome is actually quite rare and is often over diagnosed by certain imaging techniques such as MRI and CT scanning. We will discuss this later in this book when we discuss how pelvic congestion syndrome is investigated.

Non-thrombotic iliac vein lesion (NIVL)

Although May-Thurner syndrome has become the most recognised compression syndrome for the iliac veins, research from experts such as Dr Raju in the United States has shown that iliac veins can be compressed by other structures, and also on both right and left of the pelvis. In addition, there can be vestigial valves (i.e. valves that have never formed properly that are probably there from evolutionary times) that can act as narrowings in the iliac veins.

These things that can cause narrowing of the iliac veins but are not the results of a previous DVT are called "non-thrombotic iliac vein lesions" (NIVL).

Fortunately, these things appear to be uncommon as causes of pelvic congestion syndrome. However, once again they can exist and cause problems, and so we will consider them later in the chapter where we discuss investigation by imaging.

Venous stasis

Of the three venous mechanisms that might be involved in some cases of pelvic congestion syndrome, I have left venous stasis to the last. Just to remind you, the first two were venous reflux and venous obstruction.

It is probably incorrect to leave venous stasis to the last of the three from the point of view of importance. As we will discuss later, venous stasis is probably much more important than we have previously thought in understanding why venous disease causes pain and inflammation. Without doubt, venous stasis in the legs is a major cause of skin damage and venous leg ulceration as discussed in my book "Leg Ulcer Treatment Revolution". Increasingly, research suggests that it may well be a major, if not the major, cause of the pain and aching felt in pelvic congestion syndrome and the associated chronic pelvic pain due to pelvic venous disorders.

So what is venous stasis and how can it cause inflammation?

Simply, venous stasis means very slow-moving blood in the veins. This movement might not even be forward but may be a shunting of the blood back and forth. However, the blood in venous stasis cannot be completely stationary, as blood will clot if it does not move at all. Therefore, blood in venous stasis is moving just enough so that it does not clot. However, it is sitting in veins, and is not being pumped back to the heart.

As discussed earlier, venous blood transports the waste products from tissues and organs back to the liver, heart and kidneys. Arterial blood is full of oxygen and nutrients. These are used by the organs and tissues. Hence venous blood is full of carbon dioxide and the waste products of metabolism such as urea. In newspapers and many popular magazines these are often called "toxins" although this is not strictly accurate.

Fig 23

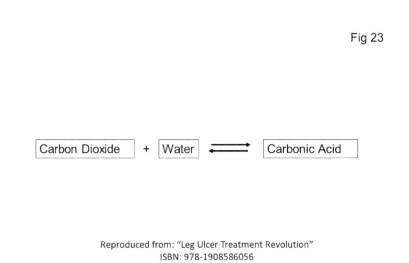

Reproduced from: "Leg Ulcer Treatment Revolution"
ISBN: 978-1908586056

Figure 23: Chemical reaction showing that carbon dioxide dissolving in water forms carbonic acid. This is a reversible reaction.

Carbon dioxide dissolves in water to form carbonic acid (Figure 23). As blood is predominantly water, the carbon dioxide dissolves in this water making the venous blood acidic. Not surprisingly, acidic blood starts irritating the vein wall and causing inflammation. This irritation and inflammation are enhanced by any other waste products that are also in the venous blood.

Normally this blood would be flushed back to the heart and from there to the lungs, liver and kidneys. The lungs would get rid of the carbon dioxide and replace it with oxygen, and the liver and kidneys get rid of urea and the other waste products of metabolism.

Fig 24

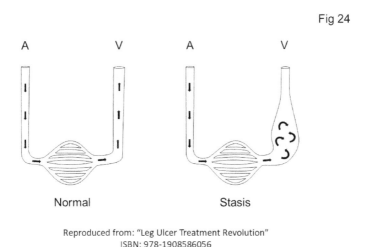

Figure 24: Diagram showing the difference between normal blood flow through the capillaries (left) and the effects of venous stasis (right).

However, in venous stasis, the venous blood remains in the veins (Figure 24). The red blood cells and white blood cells in the blood are living cells. As such, they continue to metabolise, using any available oxygen left in the venous blood and producing even more carbon dioxide and waste products. Therefore, the blood in venous stasis continues to get even more acidic and cause even more inflammation of the venous walls the longer it stays in the veins.

Although we are not talking about treatments yet, it should already be fairly clear that clearing venous stasis out of veins would be a very good idea. We will come back to this later.

Now we have considered venous reflux, venous obstruction and venous stasis, we can start to look at the symptoms and signs that patients with pelvic congestion syndrome suffer from.

Chapter 5

The Symptoms and Signs of Pelvic Congestion Syndrome

If you have been reading this book in order, up until this point we have looked at the veins in the pelvis, how they work and what can go wrong with them.

This chapter looks at what symptoms and signs patients get from pelvic congestion syndrome. Before we launch into these symptoms and signs, it is worth looking at the term "pelvic congestion syndrome" itself.

Pelvic congestion syndrome as a diagnosis

When we were working on the international guidelines for pelvic congestion syndrome which were published in August 2019, one of the first things that was noted was that the term "pelvic congestion syndrome" is probably one of the worst medical terms around.

Of course, in one way, it does make sense. Syndrome means a collection of signs or symptoms that can vary depending on presentation. Congestion means that the tissue or organ in question is full of blood and is under pressure - in this case the veins of the pelvis are full and under pressure. Pelvic is self-explanatory.

The problem with pelvic congestion syndrome as a diagnosis is that it covers such a diverse number of conditions from pelvic pain, hip pain, veins in the intimate areas of both sexes and even leg varicose veins. However, no one so far has been able to come up with a better name that has met wide approval.

Several workers in the field of pelvic veins want to change the name from pelvic congestion syndrome (PCS) to pelvic venous disorder (PVeD). However, as we will discuss later, many patients who come to see us with classic symptoms of pelvic congestion syndrome are found not to have any venous cause for their symptoms. If we change the name to pelvic venous disorders, this would clearly be a problem for such patients.

As such, in the short term, it seems sensible to make a clinical diagnosis of pelvic congestion syndrome if a patient has classic symptoms and signs of pelvic congestion, and then confirm that this pelvic congestion syndrome is due to pelvic venous disorder, if a venous disorder is identified to be the likely cause. Of course, there is a further problem that we will discuss later, where some patients have both pelvic congestion syndrome symptoms and have pelvic venous reflux identified, but the venous problem is not actually causing the symptoms. This is probably getting a bit too deep for this stage in the book, and so we will return to it later.

As such we are stuck with pelvic congestion syndrome as a label at the moment and have to explain to patients with these diverse symptoms or signs that all of them can be part of the same condition.

Conversely, many of the symptoms and signs of pelvic congestion syndrome can also be caused by other conditions. Back pain can be caused by a bad back. Pelvic pain by endometriosis or infection. Leg varicose veins can just be leg varicose veins. Therefore, I am sure that in future years there will be much better terms for these different conditions and much better classifications. However, at the present time, we can only go forward with our current understanding.

"Hysterical women"

I have always found it interesting how doctors and nurses accept easily the presence of pelvic venous reflux in males presenting with varicose veins around the testicle (varicocele) and associated aching because they can see the problem, but completely ignore women with chronic aching in the pelvis.

As we saw previously, apart from the fact the ovary is on the inside and the testicle on the outside, the venous anatomy is virtually identical. In general terms, for every male with a varicocele, there is a woman with a ovarian varicocele hidden in her pelvis.

It is common to several different conditions that many, if not most, doctors and nurses seem to find it very hard to accept symptoms when they cannot see anything that is obviously wrong.

It is an interesting aside that the term "hysterical" has its derivations from "hysterika", the Greek word for the womb. Although this is often attributed to the idea that women show excessive emotion because they have a womb, I suspect that it is also partially due to the lack of understanding in the past of pelvic congestion syndrome. We have been involved in compiling a report on the prevalence of pelvic congestion syndrome in the UK. Using a freedom of information act, it was found that 13 - 40% of women going to gynaecologists with chronic pelvic pain had pelvic congestion syndrome ("The Impact of Pelvic Congestion Syndrome" 2017).

However, as most gynaecologists do not recognise this as a diagnosis, nor put patients forward for treatment of their venous reflux, these patients end up being misdiagnosed with endometriosis or being told there was nothing wrong with them or being referred to pain clinics or even psychiatrists. Using these figures, this suggests that even in the UK, between 500,000 and 1,500,000 women are affected in this way.

With this prevalence of pelvic discomfort or pain, which goes undiagnosed and untreated, it would not be surprising if the word hysterical had become commonly used due to the number of women complaining of such symptoms and being disbelieved.

My classification of pelvic congestion syndrome

Over the years that I have been presenting to international conferences on this subject, I have developed a simple classification that I use. This is based on what the patient feels (symptoms) and what can be seen (signs). These are then separated into the different anatomical areas that each are found in.

As our understanding of pelvic congestion syndrome increases, more and more conditions are fitting into this framework. However so far, this framework still encompasses pelvic congestion syndrome and helps people understand how it can present (Figure 25).

My classification of pelvic congestion syndrome is split into:

1 - Symptoms:
>> A: Symptoms inside the pelvis
>> B: Symptoms outside the pelvis
2 - Signs:
>> A: Signs seen on the pelvis / lower abdomen
>> B: Signs seen on the legs

Fig 25

Whiteley PCS Classification

Presentation of Pelvic Congestion Syndrome (PCS):

>> 1 – Symptoms:

>>> A – Inside pelvis
>>> B – Outside pelvis

>> 2 – Signs:

>>> A – Seen on pelvis / lower abdomen
>>> B – Seen on legs

Figure 25: The Whiteley Classification on Pelvic Congestion Syndrome – a simple way to order the symptoms and signs of this condition.

1A - Symptoms inside the pelvis

The symptoms inside the pelvis that patients with pelvic congestion syndrome due to venous courses complain about, include general symptoms affecting the whole of the lower abdomen and pelvis or specific structures within the pelvis itself.

General pelvic pain or "dragging". Many patients complain of a dragging or aching discomfort, sometimes bad enough to be called chronic pelvic pain (CPP). This is worse when the patient is sitting or standing and is improved when the patient is lying flat or even lying down with their bottom elevated. If you have read the last chapter, you will understand that lying down and elevating the bottom will not only stop venous reflux but will also empty the stasis blood from any dilated veins.

Sometimes this pain is found on one side or the other. Medically we call the lower abdomen on the right and left, the right iliac fossa and the left iliac fossa respectively. Therefore, chronic pelvic pain can sometimes be localised to the left or right iliac fossa or sometimes just the whole of the lower abdomen.

The rectum and lower colon are also in the pelvis. Inflammation of this part of the bowel from pelvic venous problems can cause the symptoms of irritable bowel syndrome.

Because the bladder also sits in the pelvis, the irritation caused by the pelvic veins in pelvic congestion syndrome can also cause an irritable bladder.

Of course, both irritable bowel syndrome and an irritable bladder can have other causes, and this is one of the problems with diagnosing pelvic congestion syndrome as pelvic venous disorder without a specialist scan.

On the other hand, it is surprising how many patients who have had treatment for their pelvic venous reflux as part of their treatment for vulvar or leg varicose veins, find that their irritable bowel or irritable bladder has improved or even resolved completely.

One of the major internal pelvic symptoms of pelvic congestion syndrome in women is a deep pain or discomfort during or after sexual intercourse. Once again, this is due to the vagina being within the pelvis and surrounded by the veins affected by pelvic congestion syndrome. Hence this discomfort is usually deep rather than superficial or around the entrance of the vagina. Although it can happen during sexual intercourse, it often occurs as a deep ache afterwards as well. This can be so severe that it can stop women having a normal sex life.

Looking at the symptoms above, and just as we have already noted with irritable bowel syndrome and an irritable bladder, it is clear that other conditions can cause the same range of symptoms.

At the moment general practitioners, gynaecologists, as well as other doctors and nurses treating such women, look for all other causes of the symptoms first.

Once they have exhausted the usual diagnoses, patients with pelvic congestion syndrome are usually either misdiagnosed, and therefore get inappropriate or even ineffective treatment, or are discharged without a positive diagnosis. In these cases, patients are frequently left to try and find a diagnosis for themselves.

In the future, it might be more cost-effective and sensible for women who have the symptoms and signs of pelvic congestion syndrome to have a transvaginal venous duplex ultrasound scan performed using the Holdstock-Harrison protocol, which will often find a diagnosis with far less expense or risk of complications than many other investigations currently used for chronic pelvic pain and other associated symptoms. This is particularly true with invasive surgery such as diagnostic laparoscopy.

1B - Symptoms outside the pelvis

It may seem strange that veins inside the pelvis can cause symptoms outside of the pelvis. However, it is well documented that patients with pelvic congestion syndrome often have pain low in their back. It is often a dull ache that is quite unremitting when sitting or standing, but generally improves with lying down, even if it does take some hours for the improvement to be felt.

It is also possible for female patients to get pain or aching in the vulva and labia or indeed the perineal area. In males, varicoceles cause an aching in the affected scrotum. Some males also have been documented as having discomfort in the perineal area.

In 2016, two of my patients underwent treatment for leg varicose veins caused by pelvic venous reflux (2B below). They happened to have hip pain and had been told by their doctors that they had osteoarthritis in the hips and may need hip replacement sometime in the future. In both cases, the hip pain completely disappeared after treatment of the pelvic venous reflux that was causing the pelvic congestion syndrome.

This appears to be the first report of pelvic congestion syndrome causing hip pain. However, with the current increasing interest in pelvic congestion syndrome, we suspect that more such cases will be reported and, indeed, other symptoms outside of the pelvis may also come to light.

One further symptom that can be classed as "outside the pelvis" in males is that erectile dysfunction has also been associated with pelvic congestion syndrome. Recently a surgeon from Singapore called Sriram Narayanan has been curing some males with impotence by treating pelvic veins using a very simple local anaesthetic procedure to block off pelvic varicose veins.

2A - Signs seen on the pelvis / lower abdomen

In medicine, when something can be seen rather than felt, it is called a sign. The signs of pelvic congestion syndrome that are seen on the pelvis are all different sorts of varicose veins seen bulging the skin in different areas of the pelvis.

The commonest of these are probably haemorrhoids. Both sexes get haemorrhoids and published research from The Whiteley Clinic shows a strong correlation between haemorrhoids and reflux in the internal iliac veins.

In women, particularly after childbirth (although also seen in women who have not had children), varicose veins of the labia, vulva and vagina are relatively common. Although these can often be relatively small, in some patients they can be large and very embarrassing. I have had patients in whom the vulval varicose veins are so large they are unable to pass urine properly, wear bikinis or swimsuits and are too embarrassed to have intimate relationships. Fortunately, these can all be cured with the techniques we have developed at The Whiteley Clinic.

In men, the same veins are seen as either varicoceles (veins around the testicles) or less commonly as varicose veins of the scrotum itself.

In both sexes, although very uncommonly, there can be varicose veins of the perineum and varicose veins extending up onto the buttocks (Figure 26).

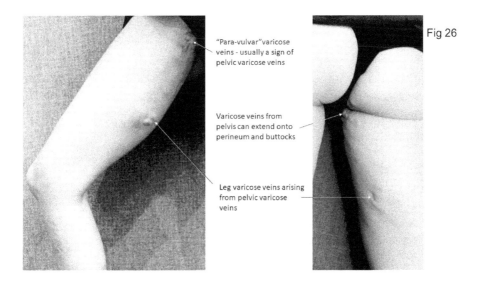

"Para-vulvar" varicose veins - usually a sign of pelvic varicose veins

Varicose veins from pelvis can extend onto perineum and buttocks

Leg varicose veins arising from pelvic varicose veins

Fig 26

Figure 26: Picture of female patient with leg varicose veins from pelvic origin (2B signs). There are varicose veins on legs, in the upper inner thighs ("para-vulvar") and in the perineum, ascending onto the buttocks.

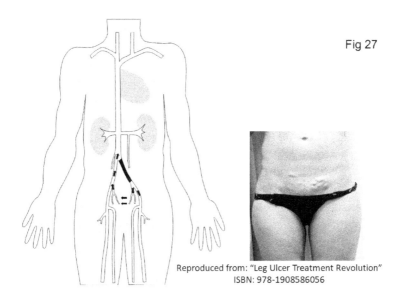

Fig 27

Reproduced from: "Leg Ulcer Treatment Revolution"
ISBN: 978-1908586056

Figure 27: Picture of a patient with varicose veins running across the lower abdomen above the pubic area (2B signs). These veins, and veins running up the flanks, indicate obstructed veins in the pelvis. This is a serious sign and needs investigating.

Finally, although rarer, there is a very important sign on the pelvis that needs to be noted. If there is a blockage of one or more of the iliac veins, then varicose veins can be seen dilated on the lower abdomen or up the flanks (Figure 27). This is a very serious sign as it shows the complete blockage of the iliac veins or even the inferior vena cava.

2B - Signs seen on the legs

Pelvic congestion syndrome contributes to leg varicose veins in a surprisingly high number of patients. Venous reflux in pelvic varicose veins (pelvic congestion syndrome) can escape from the pelvis and into the leg veins by several routes. Vein specialists have named these pelvic "escape points", although experts argue as to how many there are. Reports range from 4 to 7 escape points.

Regardless of how many escape points there may be academically, what is most important for the patient is to understand that leg varicose veins can arise from pelvic varicose veins. In other words, pelvic congestion syndrome can cause leg varicose veins as can be seen in Figure 26.

The Whiteley Clinic has been at the forefront of this research. We have shown that 1 in 6 women with leg varicose veins have a significant part of their leg varicose veins arising from pelvic varicose veins (pelvic congestion syndrome). Usually these veins appear on the inside of the upper thigh, next to the vulva (Figure 26). We have also shown that in such women, failure to identify these pelvic varicose veins and treat them, is one of the major reasons that women get varicose veins back again after varicose vein treatment of their legs.

Not surprisingly, as most doctors who treat varicose veins are not vein specialists but are vascular surgeons who specialise in arteries, general surgeons, radiologists or other doctors who do not specialise in veins, most patients with varicose veins only have their leg veins checked and treated. As such, the one in six patients whose veins are actually arising from the pelvis are not treated adequately and so their varicose veins often recur very quickly.

It is for this reason that every patient who is assessed for leg varicose veins at The Whiteley Clinic has a careful duplex looking for veins coming into the leg from the pelvis. If any of these veins are found, the patient is then offered a specialist transvaginal venous duplex ultrasound scan performed using the Holdstock-Harrison protocol.

Recently, we have also shown the same in 1 in 30 men. Again, we have found that these men have often had varicose vein surgery by vascular surgeons (who specialise in arteries), general surgeons or interventional radiologists, who do not specialise in venous disorders, and so no attention has been paid to the pelvic veins at all. As such, the varicose veins have come straight back again after treatment as the pelvic vein reflux was left untreated.

In the past, we have thought that varicose veins arising from the pelvis and descending into the legs were probably only related to minor varicose veins and not more severe conditions.

However, we have recently seen patients with severe skin damage around their ankles totally due to pelvic congestion syndrome and pelvic varicose veins communicating with leg veins. We have also published one case of a venous leg ulcer being formed the same way. This patient was part of our male pelvic vein study. In these cases, treatment of the pelvic congestion syndrome completely cured the patient, and the usual veins in the legs that cause varicose veins (great and small saphenous veins) were left alone as they were completely normal. Only the visible surface veins on the legs needed treatment once the pelvic venous reflux had been cured.

As such, any doctor or nurse assessing or treating leg varicose veins should fully understand pelvic congestion syndrome and be able to investigate and treat it. Patients with varicose veins who go to doctors who do not look for or treat pelvic congestion syndrome will clearly have a very much higher chance of recurrent varicose veins again after treatment.

How pelvic congestion syndrome causes symptoms and signs

There has been considerable interest in the research world recently to try and work out why pelvic venous congestion causes chronic pelvic pain as well as the other 1A and 1B symptoms (symptoms inside the pelvis and symptoms outside of the pelvis).

A recent review of all of the world literature in this area has come up with several possible causes.

Engorgement of the veins. The venous reflux stretches the vein walls and by dilating the veins, causes venous stasis. These factors can stimulate pain receptors in the vein wall causing pelvic pain.

Release of neurotransmitter from the vein wall. There are several neurotransmitters that have been suggested as culprits and blocking these with certain drugs can help relieve some of the pain.

Mechanical pressure. The dilated veins can press on structures in the pelvis causing pain by direct pressure on them.

At the most basic level, we know that the final result of venous disorders is inflammation. This is true whether the venous disorders cause venous reflux with blood falling the wrong way down the veins due to valve failure, venous obstruction where the blood cannot flow normally back to the heart, or venous stasis where blood stagnates, moving just enough to stop clotting, but becoming acidic and irritating the vein walls.

However, when it comes to advising patients on treatment, it becomes less important to know the exact mechanism of how the symptoms occur. What is important to know is that if we stop any venous reflux, relieve any venous obstruction and remove any venous stasis, the symptoms improve or disappear.

The same can be said for the signs of pelvic venous disorder, 2A (varicose veins visible around the pelvis and lower abdomen) and 2B (varicose veins of the legs).

Once again, we know that venous reflux disorder is generally ascending in nature. However, the mechanism of why veins become varicose when venous reflux has become established, is due to the column of blood falling down the incompetent vein by gravity. The impact of the column of blood falling down the main vein stretches the walls of the tributaries and these become varicose (dilated). In the legs there is a second sort of reflux called active reflux (or diastolic reflux) but there is no evidence that this is present in pelvic venous disorder.

It used to be thought that it was venous pressure that stretches the vein walls. However, it is more likely that it is the impact of the column of blood falling down the vein that does the stretching. Long periods of standing or sitting still without movement will stop the normal pumping of venous blood back towards the heart and will further worsen any varicosities. Of course, this also worsens any damage due to associated venous stasis.

The principles of venous reflux are to stop all of the reflux from the most proximal extent to the most distal extent, leaving only the veins that are competent and can pump blood back to the heart. We will come onto the exact ways that we can achieve this in the pelvic veins in a later chapter.

When visible varicose veins are present because of obstruction due to the main veins being either blocked or compressed, the visible veins are bypassing the high resistance area that is obstructed or compressed. Therefore, the treatment is to relieve the obstructed vein, allowing blood to start flowing normally again. This will take the pressure out of the varicose veins and, if they do not disappear, they can then be treated safely as they are not needed as bypasses.

Finally, venous stasis does not cause visible varicose veins. The treatment of venous stasis is part of the treatment of the symptoms, rather than the treatment of any visible signs externally.

Now that we have a good understanding of the anatomy of the pelvic veins, how they function, what can go wrong with them and, when they do go wrong, what symptoms and signs occur, we can consider how we should investigate and identify the venous pathology. In simple terms, we are now going to look at how we investigate pelvic congestion syndrome.

Chapter 6

Investigations for Pelvic Congestion Syndrome

How patients with pelvic congestion syndrome present to doctors

Before we launch into investigations, it is worth recapping which patients have got pelvic congestion syndrome and so how they might present to a doctor.

As we have already discussed earlier in the book, patients with pelvic congestion syndrome can present with widely different symptoms or signs. Those who have got symptoms alone, either inside the pelvis (1A) or outside of the pelvis (1B) have often been through months or even years of investigations. They have often seen multiple different generalists and specialists, and often have become very disillusioned about ever finding a cause for their symptoms. Worse still, some have had the chronic pains for so long that even when the underlying cause is found and treated, the pain is not completely resolved. It has become a learned pathway in the brain.

In addition, as we have already mentioned, some patients with clear symptoms of pelvic congestion syndrome end up having a completely normal transvaginal duplex ultrasound using the Holdstock-Harrison protocol, and so have the symptoms of pelvic congestion syndrome but of non-venous origin. Thus, until a duplex scan is done, no one with symptoms alone (1A and/or 1B) should be diagnosed with pelvic venous disorder (PVeD).

Patients who have got the signs associated with pelvic congestion syndrome are somewhat easier to diagnose. Most patients with signs around the pelvis and lower abdomen (2A) have got underlying venous causes for the signs and so it is much safer to give them a label of pelvic venous disorder (PVeD) even before a definitive scan has been performed.

However, we do see many patients with varicose veins around the vulva, varicose veins extending onto the buttocks and haemorrhoids who do not have significant pelvic venous reflux. Indeed, although we know there is a link between pelvic venous reflux and haemorrhoids, if haemorrhoids are the only problem, it would be wrong to start investigating the other pelvic veins if there were no other symptoms or signs that needed addressing.

When considering patients with 2A signs, it is worth noting that these do fall into two quite distinct patterns. Varicose veins running across the front of the lower abdomen, usually just above the pubic bone, or varicose veins running up the flanks, are indicative of obstructive pelvic vein problems as these are acting as external bypasses. We could subdivide these as 2AO (the "O" for obstructive).

The 2A varicose veins seen in the vagina, vulva, labia, perineum, around the buttocks, haemorrhoids and around the testicles in men are almost always due to venous reflux. As such, it could be possible to assign these 2AR (the "R" is for reflux). However, there may be occasional cases where the veins are due to nutcracker or May-Thurner, and so I do not use this classification yet, unless a scan has been performed and obstruction confirmed or refuted.

The easiest of all patients with pelvic congestion syndrome are those who present with leg varicose veins and, on examination, are found to have varicose veins in the para-vulvar region (on the upper inner thigh next to the vulva - Figure 26) or with varicose veins passing diagonally down the back of the thighs. These patients with 2B signs, usually have pelvic varicose veins that need treatment to reduce the risk of leg varicose veins recurring in the future.

Finally, patients can have more than one presentation. It is quite usual for us to see patients with leg varicose veins arising from the pelvis (2B) who have no idea that their varicose veins might be linked to pelvic veins. When we examine them and find that veins are coming from the pelvis, they quite often volunteer that they have pelvic symptoms either internally (1A) or externally (1B) and have either never had them investigated, or have had them investigated and no one has been able to find a cause. These patients are usually very happy when they get both their leg varicose veins treated as well as get an improvement in their pelvic symptoms, at the same time.

An even more fascinating group of patients are those that turn up with leg varicose veins arising from the pelvis (2B) and absolutely no pelvic symptoms at all. When they have their pelvic veins treated as part of the leg varicose veins treatment, they frequently say that their pelvic symptoms have improved considerably, even though they did not have pelvic symptoms at presentation. One lady in this position even said it was like having a "facelift of her pelvis".

The simple explanation for this is that when low-level pains have been present for a very long time, they often become part of a person's psyche, and become accepted by as "normal" by the patient. It is a bit like wearing an uncomfortable or itchy shirt. If you have had it on all day, you forget that it is uncomfortable. It is only when you take it off and get the relief that you realise how itchy it was.

Therefore, having run through these different possible presentations of pelvic congestion syndrome, we can now consider which investigations are useful to make the diagnosis.

You might be quite surprised that some of the investigations that are most widely used are in fact quite inaccurate and probably should not be trusted to give an accurate diagnosis.

What are we looking for?

Unless a patient has clear signs of obstructed pelvic veins (varicose veins running across the lower abdomen just above the pubic area, or varicose veins running up the flanks - 2AO signs as above) then the first thing we are looking for is the presence of pelvic vein reflux in the gonadal veins or the internal iliac veins. We can look for an obstructive cause for any reflux later as we know this is much rarer and is unlikely to be present if there is no obvious reflux in any of the pelvic veins, nor obvious dilated varicose veins in the pelvis.

We have shown that venous reflux is an ascending problem in both the leg veins and the gonadal veins, and so therefore we need to know if there is reflux in the lower part of the gonadal veins. The internal iliac veins are already low in the pelvis and so any investigation looking at the lower end of the gonadal veins is also going to be in the same area as the internal iliac veins.

This is important as our research has shown that the commonest pattern of pelvic vein reflux is reflux in the left ovarian vein and both internal iliac veins (Figure 19). Hence any investigation that does not include looking for reflux in the internal iliac veins is virtually useless.

Finally, we are looking for venous reflux. As we have seen in earlier chapters, reflux in the pelvic veins is a passive reflux, with the blood refluxing down incompetent veins by gravity. Therefore, any test that is performed with a patient lying flat is not going to show reflux in an incompetent vein. Although artificial manoeuvres might be incorporated to try and stimulate such reflux, there will clearly be errors in either over diagnosing or under diagnosing the problem, as this is not the normal physiological situation.

Therefore, from first principles it is clear that we need a test that can:

- visualise the bottom of the gonadal veins in the pelvis

- visualise the internal iliac veins in the pelvis

- be performed with the patient either upright or at a steep

"head-up" angle so reflux will occur in incompetent veins

- accurately diagnose venous reflux

In the past, before the function of the pelvic veins was well understood, radiologists produced guidelines in research papers as to the "normal diameter" of pelvic veins. Most of the research concentrated on the gonadal veins as these were thought to be the only important pelvic veins associated with reflux. Amazingly, many doctors still feel this is the case!

Because radiologists tend to use CT scanning, MRI (often called MRV when used for veins) and venography for veins deep within the body and pelvis, they produced guidelines that suggested that a measurement of the diameter of the gonadal vein could be used to determine normal from abnormal.

It is common for radiologists to use a cut-off of either 6mm diameter or 8mm diameter as a "normal" diameter for a gonadal vein. What this means is if a patient has a CT scan MRV or venography and are lying flat, and their gonadal vein is measured to be one of these diameters or more, it is diagnosed as "abnormal". If it is less, it is diagnosed as "normal".

To a vein expert such as myself, this is clearly ridiculous. In the 1990s it was well known amongst venous specialists that the size of a vein in the leg was irrelevant when assessing reflux associated with varicose veins or leg ulcers. After all, larger people tend to have larger veins and smaller people have smaller veins. In addition, exercise, body habitus and many other factors including position, temperature and anxiety also play a part. It was proven that any diameter measurement was useless, and the only relevant investigation was to use duplex ultrasound scanning to look for venous reflux to diagnose if the vein was incompetent or not.

Because duplex ultrasound uses the Doppler principle, the ultrasound can accurately show blood flow in veins, not only measuring which direction the blood is flowing but also how fast.

In order to see reflux in the saphenous veins in the leg, patients had to be standing with the weight on the other leg or on a table that tilted so they were in a severe head up position. Lying flat was useless as there was no gravity to cause the blood to reflux. Although this was all proven in the 1990s, I have recently been involved in a case where a German surgeon working in England was still scanning his patients for varicose veins when they were lying flat! Fortunately, such terrible practices are quite rare now.

However, it is shocking that despite all of these lessons we learnt in the 1990s, and all of the research papers and textbooks that have been published with regards investigating varicose veins and venous reflux in the saphenous veins in the legs, this is all ignored by interventional radiologists and surgeons who are now becoming interested in pelvic congestion syndrome and pelvic venous disorders. Whether, it is because they do not come from a true venous background, or whether it is because the pelvic veins are deep inside the body and so therefore, they regard them somehow as having completely different physiology, is unclear to me.

In order to prove the point, we performed a research study that we published five years ago measuring the diameter of ovarian veins in ladies with and without ovarian vein reflux. We found that there was absolutely no correlation between the presence of reflux and diameter. There were big and small veins that showed venous reflux, and big and small veins of the same sizes that showed no reflux. Our study showed that if diameter of the vein was used to determine treatment, half of the veins that were treated would be normal and not need treatment, and conversely half of the veins that would be left untreated because they were "normal", were actually refluxing!

It is probably not surprising that many research studies looking at the success or failure of symptom relief after pelvic vein treatments only tend to show a 70-80% success rate from treatment.

Until we can get everybody using the same diagnostic criteria and the same tests, based on science, logic and research, it will be almost impossible to compare results and make sense of treatment strategies between different hospitals and clinics.

Having explained the principles, we are now going to look at the tests that are usually used to investigate pelvic congestion syndrome, particularly if a diagnosis of pelvic vein reflux is being entertained.

Common investigations for pelvic congestion syndrome

The common investigations for chronic pelvic pain or other pelvic symptoms in women, and sometimes men, are:

- Laparoscopy

- Venography

- Magnetic resonance imaging/magnetic resonance venography

(MRI/MRV)

- Computerised tomography (CT scanning)

- Transabdominal duplex ultrasound scanning

- Transvaginal duplex ultrasound scanning

Laparoscopy

Although laparoscopy is quite rightly called "keyhole" surgery or "minimally invasive" surgery, it still is surgery. The insertion of a laparoscope into the abdominal cavity requires a general anaesthetic and admission to an operating theatre. There is a very small risk of perforation of the bowel or something else within the abdomen. The cost of the surgeon, anaesthetist, nurses and facility is considerable. Although laparoscopy can tell whether there is an ovarian tumour, adhesions, a lump of endometriosis, infection or some other conditions, it cannot diagnose pelvic congestion syndrome.

This is because in laparoscopy, the laparoscope is introduced into what is called the "peritoneal cavity". This is a cavity lined with a layer called peritoneum. Although it is possible to see the stomach, liver, gallbladder, spleen, small intestine, uterus, ovaries and bladder, it is not possible to see anything much that lies behind the peritoneal layer.

Moreover, in order to get the laparoscope into the abdomen, gas is pumped into the abdominal cavity to make room for the laparoscope. This gas will tend to pressurise venous blood out of veins in the abdomen and pelvis.

The pelvic veins lie on the other side of the peritoneal layer at the back of the abdomen and under the lowest part of the peritoneum in the pelvis. Therefore, although veins might be glimpsed in some patients through this thin membrane, particularly if they are very slim, there can be no assessment of venous reflux. Therefore, the very best that can be achieved with laparoscopy is to exclude other causes for pelvic pain or symptoms and to say whether there are obvious varicose veins in the pelvis. Failure to see them on laparoscopy is not enough to say that they are not present.

Therefore, if pelvic congestion syndrome from pelvic venous reflux is suspected, it would make much more sense to use a far cheaper investigation such as transvaginal venous duplex ultrasound to look for pelvic congestion syndrome first, saving patients the time, risks and expense of laparoscopy if a positive diagnosis was found by duplex.

Venography

To a non-medical person, venography sounds like the ideal investigation to look for abnormal veins.

Venography is the injection of a contrast fluid (commonly but incorrectly called a "dye") into the veins, and then taking x-rays to see where it flows. However, there are many problems with this investigation for pelvic congestion syndrome.

X-rays are ionising radiation and nowadays should only be used if there is no other alternative. Contrast fluid (or more correctly contrast medium) is much denser than blood and therefore does not flow the same way that blood flows naturally in the veins. If the contrast flows in a vein, then it can be seen on x-ray. But if the contrast does not flow into a vein, even though blood may be flowing in it, it will not be seen by the venogram. Therefore, it is possible to miss veins by assuming that the x-ray contrast seen on the x-ray screen is mimicking blood.

Venograms are usually performed lying flat whereas varicose veins and venous reflux can only be properly investigated when the patient is either upright or at quite a severe "head-up" angle. This is a simple consequence of gravity.

Even if the patient is tipped at an acceptable angle, the contrast does not necessarily flow in the same way that venous blood does because of the difference in density. In addition, because contrast is dense and often quite viscous, it is usually injected under pressure. As we have discussed previously, even in veins where the flow can be very fast, the venous pressures are low. Contrast injected under pressure may well follow a completely different path to the surrounding blood because of the pressure that it is injected under.

When contrast is injected, it has to be injected through a long thin tube called a catheter. This catheter obviously has to be positioned somewhere. The flow of the contrast will not only depend on the pressure used to inject it through the catheter, but also on exactly where the catheter tip is placed. As we have seen previously, we have shown that the progression of reflux in the ovarian vein is an ascending pattern. Therefore, if the catheter tip is placed at the top of the vein, near the junction with the left renal vein, it is quite possible that no reflux will be seen, even though the lower half of the ovarian vein might be incompetent. An incorrect diagnosis will be made.

As such, although venography is an essential part of the treatment of pelvic congestion syndrome in most cases, it is of limited value in the diagnosis of pelvic congestion syndrome, particularly in venous reflux - which is the commonest cause.

Magnetic resonance imaging/magnetic resonance venography (MRI/MRV)

Magnetic resonance technology has transformed many areas of medicine. Being totally non-invasive and not needing any x-rays, the uses of MRI are being expanded the whole time. It can tell the difference between many different tissue types, particularly those that contain different amounts of water.

When combined with injections of contrast, veins and arteries can be seen clearly.

However, most MRI machines require the patient to lie flat. Passive venous reflux does not occur when patients lie flat. Venous reflux requires gravity.

Some radiologists are trying to get around this by making patients perform a special breathing technique called Valsalva. In this technique, the patient acts as if they are blowing out, but they keep their mouth and/or throat closed. Some doctors achieve a similar effect by getting their patients to blow out hard through a very fine straw. This raises the pressure in the chest, increasing pressure in the veins near the heart and also in the abdomen. This is done to try to stimulate reflux in incompetent veins.

Unfortunately, it does not show physiological reflux - in other words the sort of reflux that is actually present in the patient. Moreover, although the ovarian veins can be imaged with this technique with improving accuracy, the internal iliac veins cannot be seen to reflux reliably using this technique.

Published research from The Whiteley Clinic has shown that only

3% of patients we have investigated with pelvic congestion syndrome have isolated ovarian vein reflux. The other 97% have internal iliac vein reflux as all or part of their reflux pattern. As such MRI or MRV would not be useful in these patients, and indeed might well lead to a misdiagnosis and mistreatment.

More significantly, as already noted above, many doctors use the diameter of the ovarian vein, using MRV, in women to diagnose pelvic congestion syndrome. We studied this and published our results in 2015 showing that there was no correlation at all between the diameter of the ovarian vein and whether the valves were working or not. If doctors use the diameter of the ovarian vein, they will be wrong in 50% of cases.

As such, MRI/MRV is not useful as a routine investigation of pelvic congestion syndrome. It is only useful in rare cases of complex anatomy or when duplex ultrasound cannot be performed.

Computerised tomography (CT scanning)

CT scanning has little if any advantage over MRI/MRV when we are considering the investigation of pelvic congestion syndrome. It uses x-rays which are ionising radiation and we are trying to avoid this whenever possible. Patients usually lie flat which stops any proper venous reflux being identified.

Internal iliac vein reflux cannot be seen reliably and, as noted above, the diameter of the ovarian veins is also useless.

Therefore, as with MRI/MRV, CT scanning is not useful as a routine investigation for pelvic congestion syndrome. It is only useful in rare cases of complex anatomy or when duplex ultrasound cannot be performed.

Transabdominal duplex ultrasound

Duplex ultrasound is the gold standard investigation for venous reflux. It has revolutionised venous surgery since the early 1990s. Provided it is used in the right way, it provides results second to none.

Most people understand ultrasound and have seen scans of babies before birth, or other internal organs such as gallbladders. These are usually black and white images. As most people will be aware, an ultrasound is non-invasive. It is performed by putting ultrasound gel on the surface of the skin and then the ultrasound probe onto this area.

The ultrasound beams sound waves into the body and the same transducer picks up echoes, with a sophisticated computer making a picture.

Duplex ultrasound uses improved technology over and above a simple black-and-white picture, to identify any flowing blood. Using the Doppler principle, any flowing blood can be identified on the black-and-white image. It is possible to measure the velocity using a Doppler trace but this is rarely used. What most vascular technologists use is colour flow duplex ultrasound.

This is where the black-and-white picture shows all of the structures, and blood flow is superimposed on this black-and-white image as a colour map. The flowing blood can be represented in any colour, but most machines use red for flow in one direction and blue for flow in the other direction. The brightness of the colour shows the speed of the flow.

In leg varicose veins, venous duplex ultrasound has been revolutionary. Blood can be seen to flow up veins when the muscle is compressed. If the valves are working, the blood does not reflux back down the vein and so no flow is seen when the muscle is released. However, if the patient is standing and the valves are not working, blood is seen to flow up the vein on compressing the muscle, and then refluxing back down the vein on release. The ability of venous duplex ultrasonography to identify reflux in veins noninvasively has made it the gold standard test for varicose veins and venous reflux disorder in the legs.

When it comes to assessing pelvic veins, duplex ultrasound scanning can be very useful in certain areas. With skill and removing bowel gas, it can get clear images of the veins around the kidneys, and the upper parts of the gonadal veins as they pass down the back of the abdomen. In slim patients, these can be seen easier. In such patients, the gonadal veins can be seen all the way down to the top of the pelvis. In slim patients with good views, it is possible to see the gonadal veins into the pelvis and uppermost parts of the internal iliac veins. However, in larger patients, this is more difficult or even impossible.

Unfortunately, the transabdominal duplex ultrasound scan cannot see the lower ends of the ovarian veins and internal iliac veins deep in the pelvis. As explained above, 97% of the venous reflux in pelvic congestion syndrome is in the internal iliac veins, and so the inability of transabdominal duplex ultrasound to accurately see these veins, limits its use considerably. Moreover, as we know that ovarian vein reflux is an ascending problem, a competent top of the ovarian vein does not mean to say that the ovarian vein is not refluxing. As such we need to know whether the bottom end is incompetent in such cases.

Therefore, transabdominal duplex ultrasound is very useful for checking for nutcracker syndrome and May-Thurner syndrome but is not very useful for understanding what is going on in the pelvis or looking for internal iliac vein reflux. In addition, it does not show communications of pelvic vein reflux to external veins, nor the communication of internal iliac vein reflux with haemorrhoids or vulvar and vaginal varicose veins. Therefore, it is very useful when combined with transvaginal duplex ultrasound but is of limited value as a single investigation.

It should be noted at this point that investigations of pelvic vein reflux in men, or women who are unwilling or unable to have transvaginal venous duplex ultrasound, need to be by combinations of the tests above. Such combinations might be transabdominal venous duplex ultrasound and MRI, which might have to be used in conjunction with venogram as a second-best option.

It should also be noted that duplex ultrasound scanning relies totally upon the skill and experience of the person performing it. As with all techniques that rely on the operator, the accuracy of the venous duplex ultrasound scan comes down to the training of the person, their experience and how often they are performing scans. There is good evidence in many areas of life that a minimum of 5,000 hours is required to become an expert in any practical skill and 10,000 hours is probably necessary.

Many doctors who run venous clinics perform their own duplex ultrasound scans. Unfortunately, in a great many cases, this leads to misdiagnosis both in leg varicose veins as well as pelvic varicose veins. This is because they rarely perform enough scans in a day or a week to keep the expertise level high enough. Even those who use vascular technologists to perform the scans do not get better results if the vascular technologist does not perform venous scans regularly. A great many vascular technologists specialise in arteries and only do a few venous cases scattered throughout the week.

As such, The Whiteley Protocol demands that all of our scans are performed by vascular technologists fully trained in The Whiteley Protocol (which is our general approach to venous conditions of the legs and pelvis) and also the Holdstock-Harrison protocol for transvaginal venous duplex ultrasonography. This protocol also now includes an abdominal component (the Holdstock-White protocol) to check for nutcracker and May-Thurner syndrome. The vascular technologists at The Whiteley Clinic have no other duties apart from venous duplex scanning every day, ensuring that their ultrasound skills are not diluted.

Transvaginal duplex ultrasound

Transvaginal duplex ultrasound scanning uses a specialist transvaginal probe, allowing the ultrasound probe to be positioned as close as possible to the internal iliac veins, their tributaries and the lower ends of the ovarian veins in the pelvis.

Judy Holdstock and Charmaine Harrison of The Whiteley Clinic spent many years in the early 2000's perfecting their protocol for investigating pelvic congestion syndrome. This has been supplemented by further work by Angie White who joined our team more recently.

The patient is placed at a 45° angle, head-up and so in an almost "sitting" position, allowing natural venous reflux to be observed due to the effect of gravity. The transvaginal ultrasound handpiece is positioned and then rotated to identify all four of the pelvic veins that are of interest. Venous reflux is checked for at rest, with the patient performing Valsalva and with the patient clenching and relaxing their buttocks - a manoeuvre called the "Kegel squeeze". This muscle contraction forces blood up the pelvic veins and then, when the muscles relax, any reflux can be identified.

All four pelvic veins - both ovarian veins and both internal iliac veins are checked in this way. Because of the position of the probe, all the tributaries can be seen, and connection of any pelvic veins with haemorrhoids, vulvar veins or leg varicose veins can also be identified.

We have published a study comparing transvaginal venous duplex ultrasound scanning using the Holdstock-Harrison protocol with diagnosis by venography, using the results of treatment for the patients as the outcome. This study, published in 2015, showed that transvaginal venous duplex ultrasonography appeared better than venography at diagnosing which veins were refluxing and needing treatment. As we used the success of treatment as the outcome, it is highly likely to be correct as getting the right result for the patient is of paramount importance.

Furthermore, Judy Holdstock and Angie White of The Whiteley Clinic have continued to develop the technique and won first prize at the American College of Phlebology in 2017. Their prize-winning research was developed from adding both transabdominal duplex of the renal veins to the Holdstock-Harrison protocol for transvaginal duplex giving a complete understanding of the whole of the pelvic venous system. Using this technique, and working on observations by Dr David Beckett, they were able to show that nutcracker syndrome rarely exists, and they were the first to describe "pseudo-nutcracker" syndrome, as we will discuss later.

As such, it is now clear that in patients who can undergo it, transvaginal venous duplex ultrasonography using the Holdstock-Harrison protocol, combined with the transabdominal investigation using the Holdstock-White protocol, is currently the gold standard investigation for pelvic congestion syndrome.

In units where there are not personnel with the skills to perform transvaginal duplex ultrasonography with these protocols, then combinations of the other tests need to be performed. However, any results must be interpreted knowing the shortcomings of each particular investigation.

Having gone through the investigations that are currently available for pelvic venous reflux, we can now mention some of the more specialist tests that can be used but are not needed in the majority of cases.

More specialised tests that can be used in pelvic congestion syndrome

As we discussed earlier in this chapter, and indeed earlier in this book, pelvic congestion syndrome covers a wide number of different conditions. Even when proven to be venous, it is possible that there can be compression or obstruction of the veins as part of the condition.

If there is any doubt following the duplex ultrasonography and other tests listed above, the following tests can be used.

Intravascular ultrasound (IVUS)

Intravascular ultrasound (IVUS) has been a major development in the vascular world. In essence, it is a tiny ultrasound probe that is situated in the tip of a long tube called a catheter, that can be passed into a blood vessel through a fine tube called a cannula.

Under local anaesthetic, a needle can be passed into the vein in the groin. A wire is passed up the needle, a dilator is passed over this and a fine plastic tube (cannula) inserted into the vein. The wire and dilator are removed. The IVUS catheter can then be passed through the cannula and into the femoral vein and up through the pelvic veins, into the inferior vena cava.

An external x-ray can be used if necessary, to check exactly where the IVUS catheter is. The catheter is then withdrawn with the ultrasound running. An image of the inside of the vein's cross-sectional area is then formed. Any compression of the vein can be seen in high resolution as a narrowing of the vein, as the catheter is pulled back through it.

Although this is "space age" stuff, it does have some drawbacks. Catheters are single use and are expensive. Moreover, investigations are usually performed with the patient lying on their back and so the significance of some narrowed areas might not be certain. In the same way that MRI/MRV and CT can often report that veins look squashed or flattened when lying flat, IVUS also sees these. The problem is that such narrowing might be positional and not significant to venous blood flow in normal activity.

Overall, IVUS gives a fantastic view of the veins and a good measurement of the cross-sectional area. It allows one to see the vein wall and can often give a good view of whatever is pushing on the vein from the outside if something is doing so. If a vein has to be stented, it can also be used after the stent has been placed, to ensure that the stent is in the right place and has had the appropriate effect on the narrowed area.

However, certainly in our own practice, we have rarely needed IVUS, and so it is a luxury to have. It is only essential in complex patients, or patients who have proven compression syndromes, who need full assessments before treating venous compressions.

Air plethysmography (APG)

Air plethysmography is a very useful and inexpensive test to measure function of the veins.

There are different protocols depending on what a doctor wants to measure. The technique that is useful for testing whether there is a significant obstruction or compression in the iliac veins, is that which has been popularised by Evi Kalodiki and Christopher Latimer.

In the simplest form, a cuff filled with air is placed around the lower leg and inflated to a certain pressure to hold it in place. The patient is told to stand and the pump filling the cuff is run until it stabilises. The patient then lies down, quickly elevating their leg. If possible, this is done on a tilt table and the patient is tilted from standing position to severe head down. If the veins in the leg and pelvis are open and there is no obstruction, the leg empties very quickly.

Conversely, if there is a narrowing or obstruction in the veins of the leg or pelvis, the flow out of the leg is impeded. This is represented by a slow deflation of the cuff (Figure 28).

Air plethysmography is an excellent screening test to look for any significant narrowing or obstruction in the pelvic veins. Although it does not show the exact position of where any such compression might be, it is inexpensive and a great functional test. If it is negative, then no expensive imaging is needed. If positive any narrowing found on subsequent imaging is known to be significant.

The alternative would be to use one of the more expensive imaging tests first. However, any compression that might be identified would still need a functional test to see whether it was significant or not.

Therefore, air plethysmography is very useful if there is any suspicion of May-Thurner, NIVL or any other iliac vein compression or obstruction.

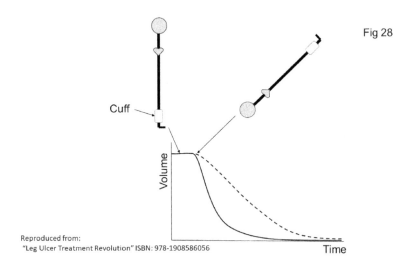

Fig 28

Cuff

Volume

Time

Figure 28: Diagram showing how air plethysmography is used to investigate possible venous outflow obstruction. A cuff around the calf measures the leg volume when standing. The patient lies down and elevates the leg (or is tipped head down on a tilt table). If the veins are open, the blood flows out quickly, reducing the leg volume rapidly (solid line). But if there is an obstruction, blood flows out more slowly (broken line).

Intra-venous pressure measurements

In arterial disease, intra-arterial pressure measurements are the gold standard investigation for a significant narrowing (stenosis). In an artery, where the blood is at high pressure and is flowing fast, any narrowing causes blood to speed up. Therefore, duplex ultrasonography, that is based on Doppler, can see this area of increased blood velocity.

However, in arteries, such a narrowing is only significant if there is a pressure drop. This is because the energy of arterial blood is measured by how much pressure there is in it. If it has to do work to get across a narrow area, then there is less energy in the blood to drive it to the tissues.

Hence the speeding up of the blood seen on duplex suggests there is a narrowing, but only pressure measurements can tell if it is truly significant.

Unfortunately, venous physiology is not the same. Venous pressures are very low and so trying to measure a drop in venous pressure over a narrowed area is very problematic. Also, veins can dilate considerably more than arteries. Hence when patients walk, not only does the flow of blood change considerably from the pumping of the leg muscles, but in addition, healthy veins can dilate. If a vein dilates, this obviously affects the velocity of the blood flowing within it.

Currently, venous pressures are measured when the patient is lying down and not moving on a x-ray table.

Protocols can overcome some of these drawbacks, but intravenous pressures do not have a major role in venous investigations now. There are some new devices such as wearable intravenous pressure monitors that might become very useful in the future. However, they are currently not available except in research units.

Now we have explained what investigations are available, we can talk about the treatments that are available for the different presentations of pelvic congestion syndrome.

Chapter 7

The Treatment of Pelvic Congestion Syndrome due to Pelvic Venous Disorders

Principles of treatment

When we come to think about the treatment of pelvic conditions, we once again have to come back to the problem that there are many different presentations and also different underlying causes for these presentations.

Therefore, to make it as simple as possible, we are going to break the treatment section down into two main areas.

In this chapter, we are going to go through the principles of treating the venous abnormalities that are found in patients presenting with pelvic congestion syndrome and are found to have a venous cause. Therefore, these patients have the diagnosis of pelvic venous disorders. Once we have discussed the principles, we will then go through the practical ways that these principles are achieved with our current treatment protocol (embodied as the pelvic vein part of The Whiteley Protocol).

In the next chapter, we will then go through the decision-making process for different patients with different presentations of pelvic congestion syndrome and different underlying problems. This should make the process of how we use the principles of The Whiteley Protocol become clearer.

So, let's start with the basic principles of treatment

Once pelvic congestion syndrome (PCS) has been suggested, and the cause of the presenting symptoms (1A, 1B) or signs (2A, 2B) has been confirmed as likely to be pelvic venous disorder (PVeD) with transvaginal venous duplex ultrasonography using the Holdstock-Harrison protocol, with the transabdominal extension using the Holdstock-White protocol, then treatment can be planned. If there is any doubt to the diagnosis, other investigations may have been ordered as in the last chapter.

However, in principle:

- in the rare cases of venous obstruction (whether complete occlusion or significant narrowing due to compression or intravenous pathology) - the obstruction needs to be treated first. Once treated, reassessment can then be made to see if any further treatment is needed for reflux.

- in most cases there is only venous reflux and so correction of this is the first priority

- venous stasis is treated at the same time as venous reflux in the majority of cases

- if there are any communications from pelvic varicose veins to significant varicose veins in the labia, vulva, vagina, perineum or legs, these are treated at the end of all other treatments.

As with all medical conditions, we need to consider conservative treatments initially, then go through medical treatments before moving on to interventional treatments. This is the standard approach in medicine following the "do no harm" principle.

However, most patients who come to see us have already been through most of the conservative and medical treatments, most commonly because that approach is part of a "shotgun approach", taken by doctors who they have consulted previously and who are unsure as to the diagnosis.

Conservative treatments

Conservative treatments in medical terms means treatments that have little or no risk. As such it usually means things that you can do or, sometimes, medications that you can take.

As we have discussed previously, pelvic congestion syndrome is usually caused by venous reflux in the gonadal and/or internal iliac veins, it can rarely be caused by venous obstruction, and whether reflux and/or obstruction, it has associated venous stasis in the pelvic veins.

As the reflux and obstruction is physical, it is unlikely that conservative treatments will have much effect, except in the most minor cases. However, it is sensible to try such conservative treatments if the symptoms or signs are not very severe and the patient is prepared to spend time and money seeing if they will work.

Position, pelvic massage and compression

Clearly from the understanding of the anatomy of the pelvic veins and how they work, as outlined in chapters 3 and 4, lying a patient flat and elevating their bottom will stop venous reflux in the pelvic veins and will also help empty venous stasis lying in dilated varicose veins in the pelvis. This is a pretty good test for pelvic congestion syndrome. There are some areas in the world where different forms of pelvic massage have also been developed, to try and keep venous stasis and reflux to a minimum.

However, in most people's day-to-day life, it is impossible to keep lying down and elevating the bottom or to keep having pelvic massage, even if it is found to work for the individual. If, however, the problem is true obstruction, then these manoeuvres are unlikely to make any difference in any case.

There has recently been a research paper published from Russia suggesting that compression pants can help. Compression pants that give compression to the vulva and perineal area, as well as compression to the anterior abdomen, seem to be able to help with the symptoms of pelvic congestion syndrome.

As many of the veins involved in pelvic congestion syndrome reside deep in the pelvis, this result is a little surprising. Moreover, pressure on the lower abdomen will also put pressure on the bladder and bowel. In some patients this may cause urinary frequency and changes in bowel habit. However, if the increase in the intra-abdominal pressure and pressure in the pelvis from compression over the front of the lower abdomen is significant, this might be a cheap and simple way to improve symptoms in some patients.

We are currently performing a randomised study at The Whiteley Clinic, supported by a research award from Bauerfeind to see if we can confirm these findings. These results should be available in 2022-2023.

As with support stockings for legs with varicose veins or other vein conditions such as leg ulcers, compression will only help whilst the compression garment is in place. As soon as it is removed, the underlying venous reflux will continue, and venous stasis accumulate. As such it is not a treatment of the condition, but a symptomatic relief whilst the garment is being worn.

Medication

Many patients use simple analgesia for any pain at home and have usually exhausted this as an option before coming for specialist treatment.

Medroxyprogesterone acetate has been used as an oral tablet with some improvement in patients with pelvic congestion syndrome proven to be due to pelvic venous reflux. This has no effect on the reflux itself but does have an effect on the neurotransmitters released as part of the inflammatory process. Therefore, this can help with symptom relief although of course it does not get to the underlying cause. As such, once again it must be recognised that this is a symptomatic relief and not a cure.

There has been some recent work on micro-purified flavonoid fraction (MPFF) which is derived from citrus fruit. This group of chemicals has been used around the world and proven to have a positive effect in the symptoms of leg varicose veins and venous leg ulcers. Largely it appears to act by reducing the inflammation caused by venous disorders. There are some interesting other possible effects that are being studied.

Once again, MPFFs can help relieve the symptoms in patients with pelvic congestion syndrome due to pelvic venous reflux and venous stasis. However, it does not cure the condition and symptoms are likely to return once the medication is stopped.

Interventional treatment for pelvic congestion syndrome due to pelvic venous disorders

When thinking of the interventional treatments, we need to separate the treatment of pelvic vein reflux causing pelvic congestion syndrome from obstruction causing the same. Stasis is common to both reflux and obstruction and so does not need specific treatment.

Research over 20 years from The Whiteley Clinic has shown that the vast majority of patients suffering from pelvic congestion syndrome (PCS) due to pelvic venous disorders (PVeD) have pelvic vein reflux as the underlying cause. Therefore, we will concentrate on the interventional treatment of pelvic vein reflux first.

Principles of venous ablation for reflux

Before proceeding to discuss interventional treatments, it is important to understand why we ablate the veins to cure patients.

Many patients worry that if we permanently close a vein, they wonder "where the blood will go". This is a common misconception and is often misunderstood even by doctors and nurses who perform venous treatments! You will often hear them say that "the blood will find another way". If you do hear that, have great concerns about the person who you are talking to!

With regards to pelvic vein reflux, we will go through the argument stepwise so that you will understand the logic of why veins need to be permanently ablated. By the end of it, you will also understand why it is essential to only ablate veins with proven reflux. That is why you should be very careful as to which test is used and why diagnosis by MRI, MRV and CT scanning alone, and even venography, is such a worry.

The first thing to consider is that veins are taking blood away from organs and back to the heart. As such, all pelvic veins should be flowing upwards (Figure 29). As we have shown before, blood would not normally flow upwards against gravity and we have already discussed in earlier chapters how blood is pumped this way. We will not repeat that, but just accept that the blood is flowing upwards against gravity.

Let us consider the simple case where the left gonadal vein in a woman has become incompetent. As she is a woman, the gonadal vein in question is the left ovarian vein. This is represented in Figure 30.

Considering the normal situation, where all of the pelvic veins are competent as in Figure 29, we can see that all of the blood entering the pelvic veins from the legs, and all of the blood emerging from the pelvic organs into the pelvic veins, will pass up the relevant pelvic veins to get to the heart. Venous blood from the legs will go up the iliac veins into the inferior vena cava straight to the heart. Venous blood from deep within the pelvis will pass up the internal iliac veins, into the common iliac veins and once again through the inferior vena cava into the heart. Venous blood from the ovaries, uterus and surrounding organs will pass up the ovarian veins, reaching the inferior vena cava (on the left via the left renal vein) and pass on to the heart.

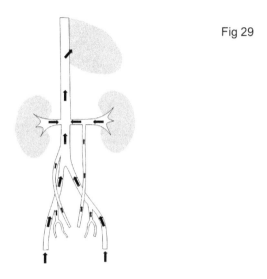

Fig 29

Figure 29: Normal direction of venous blood flow in the pelvic veins.

This is the normal situation and 100% of the venous blood from the legs and pelvis gets back to the heart.

Now let's consider the incompetent left ovarian vein with left ovarian vein reflux in Figure 30.

Once again, all the blood from the legs passes up the iliac veins and into the inferior vena cava. Most will then go on to the heart. However, some will divert into the left renal vein, refluxing down the incompetent left ovarian vein. Venous blood from the left kidney will also flow down the incompetent left ovarian vein. Venous blood from deep in the pelvis will flow up the internal iliac veins into the common iliac veins and then up the inferior vena cava.

Fig 30

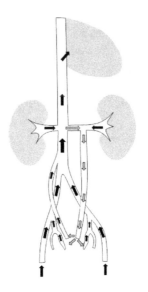

Figure 30: Left ovarian vein reflux in a woman. Blood refluxes down the left ovarian vein and into multiple tributaries in the pelvis. These dilate, becoming varicose veins in the pelvis, as the venous blood flows towards the competent veins, in order to get back to the heart.

Once again most will go back to the heart, but some can divert into the left renal vein and reflux down the left ovarian vein. Venous blood on the right side of the pelvic organs will flow up the right ovarian vein into the inferior vena cava. Once again most will go back to the heart, but some will reflux down the left ovarian vein.

As such, we can now see that although 100% of the blood starts flowing up the veins towards the heart, a certain percentage will reflux down the left ovarian vein. Let's assume this is 5%. This will mean that the heart only gets 95% of the expected blood, and 5% will fall down the left ovarian vein.

There is so much blood coming back to the heart from all the veins in the body, that the heart does not notice such a small reduction in venous blood coming back to it.

However, the reflux of blood down the left ovarian vein, which should be carrying venous blood away from the pelvis, causes dramatic effects. The refluxing blood impacts on the veins on the left side of the pelvis, stretching the walls and causing a sudden increase of pressure. This can cause inflammation and, if there is enough inflammation, this can cause pain. Moreover, the veins will dilate in the pelvis to accommodate this blood, causing venous stasis.

Obviously, this is a dynamic situation. With 5% of the blood falling back down the left ovarian vein into the pelvis, the competent veins draining the pelvis must take even more blood back to the heart. They now have to take 105% of the usual venous blood flow – ie: all of the venous blood that they have to transmit PLUS the 5% that has already been passed up the veins but has refluxed back down into the pelvis.

This refluxing blood has to go through the pelvic vein networks to be picked up through the competent pelvic veins. In this case, the internal iliac veins on both sides and the right ovarian vein, to re-join the normal route of venous blood flow from these veins (Figure 30).

So, as noted above, this now means that the internal iliac veins and right ovarian veins are not only carrying 100% of their own blood, they are having to dilate to accommodate the extra blood from the left ovarian vein reflux. In addition, the networks of veins in the pelvis get dilated (become "varicose"), due to the increased volume of blood falling down the left ovarian vein and flowing out towards these other competent veins. This is how the "pelvic varicose veins" form.

The longer this is allowed to continue, the larger the pelvic varicose veins are likely to become, the more the ovarian vein will stretch and dilate, increasing the venous reflux and the more the internal iliac veins and right ovarian vein have to work to keep up with the refluxing blood. As the pelvic varicose veins dilate, more inflammation occurs and an increasing volume of stasis blood collects in the pelvic varicose veins, increasing the chances and severity of any pelvic pain or other internal symptoms.

So, what is the logical way to treat this?

Is it logical to try to use conservative methods or drugs?

None of these methods correct the underlying problem - that is incompetence of the left ovarian vein. Indeed, if left alone, the incompetence will only worsen as the vein dilates and more blood refluxes down it, worsening the clinical situation. These conservative measures and drugs do not even stop that deterioration.

Of course, in a perfect world, we would make the left ovarian vein valves work again. This would make the left ovarian vein competent, restoring the normal function.

Unfortunately, that is impossible with currently available technology.

Therefore, the best we can currently do is to permanently block the left ovarian vein (Figure 31).

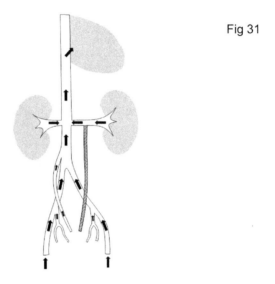

Fig 31

Figure 31: The best treatment at the current time is to permanently block the left ovarian vein, stopping the reflux. This lets all of the competent veins get back to their normal function. Now they have to transmit a little more blood than when the left ovarian vein was working normally, BUT this is far less than the amount they had to carry when they were taking all of this blood AND all of the blood refluxing down the incompetent left ovarian vein.

If we can permanently ablate this vein, the function of all the other veins return to normal. Venous blood from the left kidney can now flow through the left renal vein into the inferior vena cava without being diverted. Blood from the legs can go straight up through the iliac veins, inferior vena cava, and all of it gets to the heart. Venous blood from the deep pelvis can go up the internal iliac veins on each side, joining the blood flow from the legs, once again reaching the heart. Blood from the right ovarian vein similarly joins the inferior vena cava and reaches the heart.

Once again, order is restored and 100% of the venous blood reaches the heart.

Thus, although we have permanently ablated the left ovarian vein, we have restored the flow of venous blood back to normal without any detrimental effects to the body. In fact, we have reversed the detrimental effects to the pelvic veins and organs that were being caused by the venous reflux in the left ovarian vein.

You may think that these competent veins are now having to "work harder" to take more blood than usual, to compensate for the left ovarian vein being taken out of the system. However, the reverse is true. Once the incompetent left ovarian vein is removed, the competent veins only have to do their normal job, plus a little extra to compensate for the missing left ovarian vein. This is considerably less than this amount of blood AND all of the venous blood refluxing down the incompetent left ovarian vein.

It is important to note that this argument only holds if the correct vein has been closed (ablated).

If we had ablated a vein that was working normally (was competent) we would have worsened the situation. If we had left a vein that was incompetent untreated, again the situation would worsen with time. This is why it is so important to make sure the correct investigation has been performed and the correct treatment planned.

We see a very large number of patients at The Whiteley Clinic who have been told that they have had "pelvic vein embolisation" elsewhere, only to find that when we perform the transvaginal venous duplex with the Holdstock-Harrison protocol, either the wrong vein has been treated or it has been treated inadequately. The usual reason for this is using MRI/MRV, CT or venogram to diagnose the pelvic congestion syndrome (see previous chapter) or sometimes incorrect ablation, with the vein blocked too high and not at the bottom of the vein (see later).

How do we permanently close (ablate) a pelvic vein?

Before we discuss pelvic veins, we must review the lessons we have learnt over the last 20 years about the treatment of leg varicose veins. Just as in the chapter about imaging, lessons we have learnt in treating leg varicose veins have a direct relevance to successful treatment of the pelvic veins.

Since the 1890's, doctors had been treating leg varicose veins by open surgery. This process included cutting through the skin and superficial tissues, identifying the target vein and tying the vein with a surgical ligation.

Unfortunately, this doesn't work in the majority of cases. Usually the tie breaks down and the vein reconnects.

In the middle of the 20th century, doctors took to tying the vein and then stripping it out. The thought process was that if the vein was not just tied at one end but also stripped out, it wouldn't be able to re-connect if the ligation suture dissolved or broke. However, prize-winning research from The Whiteley Clinic in 2005, published in 2007, showed that stripping a leg vein usually results in it growing back again over time. When it grows back, we showed that it grows back again without any valves in it. Hence, when it has re-grown, it merely becomes a varicose vein once again.

In March 1999, Judy Holdstock and I performed the first endovenous surgery in the UK. Using a radiofrequency catheter, guided up the leg vein under ultrasound, we heated the vein wall to 85°C which permanently destroyed the vein. In 2004 I published the principles of how the correct amount of heat destroys a vein wall leading to permanent closure by fibrosis, and how inadequate heat will cause temporary closure by clot (thrombosis), only to reopen again when the clot resolves.

Although the early work was with radiofrequency ablation, we have subsequently shown that we can close the veins more elegantly with other methods of heating the veins. Through our research department, we have shown that different laser devices can be used to heat the vein from inside (endovenous laser ablation), and recently we have introduced microwave (endovenous microwave ablation).

In May 2019, we have introduced a totally non-invasive way of heating the veins with High Intensity Focused Ultrasound (HIFU or Echotherapy). All of these are successful because they use heat to both contract protein and to kill the cells in the vein wall. As per my hypothesis in 2004, it is the death of the cells in the vein wall that is needed to cause permanent venous ablation.

Many doctors have tried to replace this heating technique with a chemical method of injection called foam sclerotherapy. We have studied this in detail and, although foam sclerotherapy does work in small veins with thin walls, it causes clots in bigger veins with thicker walls. Because blood doesn't flow in a clotted (thrombosed) vein, it appears to have been successfully closed (ablated) on duplex ultrasound in the short term.

However, the clot slowly resolves, and the vein opens up again in the long term. Of course, when it re-opens it is still incompetent. Hence such "closure", although appearing successful in the short term, is not a permanent closure. As such a vein with a clot (thrombosis) in it is temporarily closed - but not "ablated". In legs, veins with clots in them can cause brown stains on the skin, although this is obviously not a problem with veins deep in the pelvis. However, the failure of long-term ablation is.

All the above is explained in detail in my book "Leg Ulcer Treatment Revolution".

The relevance of this explanation to the pelvic veins is that the gonadal veins and the internal iliac veins are large veins with thick walls.

As such, using the principles we have developed and proven at The Whiteley Clinic over the last 20 years, we know that the treatment of gonadal vein reflux or internal iliac vein reflux requires something akin to the heat energy from endovenous thermoablation. We also know that ultrasound guided foam sclerotherapy is insufficient and will only cause clots in the veins, which have a very high chance of re-opening at a later date.

Over the last 20 years, our continuing research has led us to produce a protocol for doctors and vascular technologists working in The Whiteley Clinic to ensure they are using the optimal methods of investigating and treating different venous disorders. Not surprisingly we call this "The Whiteley Protocol".

The Whiteley Protocol approach to the treatment of pelvic venous reflux

Because of the size of the gonadal and internal iliac veins, and the thickness of their vein walls, we would ideally like to use heat to close these veins. The smaller varicose veins in the pelvis, that are being stretched by the venous reflux from these larger veins, have thinner walls, and can be treated by foam sclerotherapy. However, if these are filled with foam sclerotherapy and the major venous reflux that has caused them is not corrected at the same time, these veins will only re-open again in the future.

Therefore, the principles are clear. We need to stop the venous reflux in the major gonadal and internal iliac veins first, and then use foam sclerotherapy in the small pelvic varicose veins including those communicating with the legs, vulva, vagina et cetera.

Unfortunately, because the gonadal veins and internal iliac veins are surrounded by sensitive structures such as arteries, ureters (the tubes from kidney to bladder that transport urine), bowel, bladder, vagina and pelvic nerves, it would be crazy to try and close these veins with heat using any of the endovenous thermal ablation devices available. Although unbelievably some doctors have tried these techniques, one can only assume that they do so because they do not understand the biology and the anatomy of the veins. It is safe to use heat in the leg veins because we can surround the veins with local anaesthetic which stops the heat from being transferred. This is called tumescence. However, we cannot do this in the pelvic veins which are deep inside the body.

Therefore, we have to permanently close (ablate) these veins using some other technique which does not require heat. There are several different techniques that have been reported. We will now go through these.

Treatments to permanently ablate refluxing pelvic veins

Embolisation with metal coils

The most widespread treatment for the ablation of incompetent pelvic veins is embolisation using metal embolisation coils. These have been designed to be placed within a vein or artery with the intention of permanently destroying it (Figure 32).

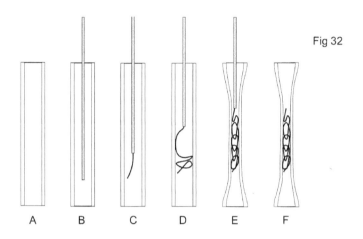

Fig 32

A   B   C   D   E   F

Figure 32: Diagram showing how embolisation coils are put into pelvic veins. A represents an incompetent section of vein to be treated. A catheter is placed into the vein (B) and when in the right place, an embolisation coil is deployed (C,D,E). As the coil emerges from the catheter it coils up, irritating the vein wall and causing spasm E. Once deployed, the catheter is removed, and the coil is embedded within the vein both by radial force of the coils and spasm of the vein wall.

Embolisation coils have been used for some 40 years or so and have a very long history to show safety within the body. They are made of metal, usually an inert metal such as platinum. Unfortunately, this does mean that they are expensive. The actual structure of the coils varies from manufacturer to manufacturer. However, the principles of how they work remain the same. They are packaged into a very fine tube called a catheter. This can be passed into a vein under x-ray control. When in position, the coil can be pushed out of the end of the catheter, where they coil up inside the vein (Figure 32). The metal coils irritate the vein wall, causing it to go into spasm. Some coils have fibres woven into them, to increase this irritation.

An additional feature of some coils is that they can be withdrawn back into the tube if the doctor is not happy with the position of the coil during this placement.

Although the coils are made out of very thin metal, when they coil, the diameter of the curve of the coil can be determined. This allows doctors to choose which size of coil diameter they wish to use. The size of the coil diameter is chosen to be much bigger than the diameter of the vein. In this way, the coil pushes hard into the vein wall and it is highly unlikely that the coil will ever move.

The biology of the interaction between the coil and the vein is very interesting and has not been fully researched at present. What is clear is that if the coil is removed soon after it is placed, then the vein comes out of spasm and can go back to being normal. However, we know that if the coil is left in place for many months, the vein is destroyed and is found to be a wisp of protein surrounding the coil. Therefore, somewhere between a few days and many months, the vein dies and becomes permanently ablated because the coil is in place.

Some patients ask if absorbable coils can be used. They like the idea that the coils are not permanent. However, this is not a good idea as it is quite like having an absorbable hip replacement! The coil is needed to keep the biological process of fibrosis going. If the coil dissolves before that process is complete, symptoms or signs will recur, and the procedure will have been thought to have failed. If that happened, either the patient would get all of the original problems back again or the risk is that the vein will re-open, and the procedure would have to be repeated.

Other patients ask if coils can be removed. Once a coil is deeply embedded and the vein has started to fibrose around it, then it is virtually impossible to remove. If this were not the case, then we would always be worried that the coils could move once inside the body.

The success rate of coil embolisation is very high and we have published our own short and long-term results showing our success rate. It is very rare for there to be a complication and in the thousands we have put in place, we have only had a couple ever move and migrate through the veins. Fortunately, these were early in our experience and with increased knowledge of how to perform the procedures, we have not seen this complication now for many years.

However, as with all procedures, it is important to get the technique exactly right and to place these coils deep down inside the vein and not leave them hanging near the top. In this situation they are both more likely to move, and also they do not treat the reflux lower in the vein. As described before, our research has shown that reflux starts from the bottom of the vein and so this is where the coil should be placed (Figure 33). This principle is the same as to whether the ovarian vein or the internal iliac vein is being embolised with the coils.

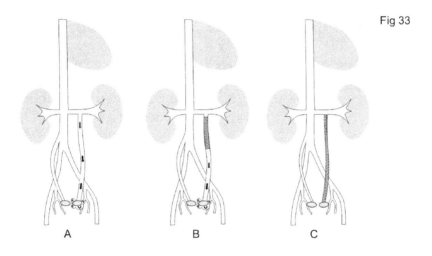

Fig 33

A   B   C

Figure 33: Left ovarian reflux (A) is often treated badly by doctors inexperienced in treating pelvic congestion, who frequently leave the embolisation coils too high in the vein (B). This increases the risk of coils moving into the main veins and then to the heart and then the lungs (embolisation) and also fails to treat the reflux lower down in the incompetent vein. Correct embolisation includes the distal part of the vein to be treated (C).

The three commonest causes of failure that we see when patients come to us having said that they have already had "coil embolisation" in other practices, are:

- The wrong veins were treated because the doctors used MRI, CT or venography and used the size of the vein to diagnose an abnormality, rather than using duplex to look for reflux

- The coils were placed too high in the vein allowing reflux to continue lower down in the vein and the varicose veins in the pelvis remain untreated

- Only the gonadal veins (ovarian in women) were treated because they are easier and longer to treat, and the actual cause of the problem from the internal iliac vein reflux was left untreated.

Finally, we have also published research showing that we have now had patients who have had coil embolisation of the pelvic veins and have subsequently got pregnant. To date all the patients going through pregnancy have had successful pregnancies with no coils moving significantly during the pregnancy nor childbirth. We have seen only one patient where a coil had moved toward the main vein during the pregnancy and so this was removed and replaced after delivery. This was a simple local anaesthetic procedure performed using the same approach as the original embolisation, as outlined below.

Technique of coil embolisation of pelvic veins

In order to get the coils into the correct veins, a thin tube or "catheter" has to be positioned exactly into the lower end of the vein to be treated. It is guided into position under x-ray control, and the procedure is performed by an interventional radiologist with experience in intravenous embolisation.

This is not a technical manual of how to do the procedure, but there is one major point that needs to be brought up. Many patients, when we start talking about coil embolisation of pelvic veins, assume that the needle will be placed in the groin. This is probably a logical assumption to a patient, as the groin is near the pelvis.

However, if you consider the anatomy of the gonadal veins and the internal iliac veins, you will see that they all run from bottom to top, with the open ends pointing upwards towards the heart.

Therefore, if the procedure was performed from the groin, there are several sharp bends that would need to be negotiated to get the catheter into place (Figure 34). When we started doing these procedures in 2000, our experience was that doctors who used the femoral approach often failed to get the coils exactly where required.

A far more sensible approach is to pass the catheter from above and directly down the vein. This is why we have always used the right jugular vein approach (Figure 34).

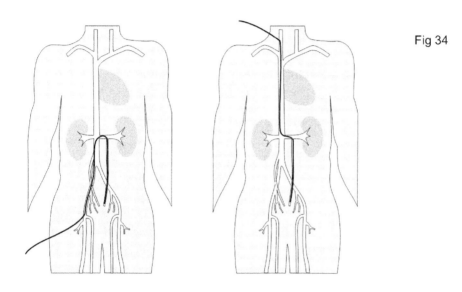

Fig 34

Figure 34: Diagram showing why we use the trans-jugular approach via the neck when performing pelvic vein embolisation. The femoral approach (left diagram) via the groin means that the catheter has to be passed up the veins, perform a "U" turn, and then be pushed back down the target vein. A much easier approach that allows far more control of positioning a catheter is the trans-jugular approach (right diagram). In this case, the catheter is more or less straight, making it far easier to control and hence more likely to get a good result for the patient.

We developed the trans-jugular approach for embolisation of the pelvic veins in 2000, and in 2014 started performing this as a walk-in, walk-out, local anaesthetic procedure in our clinic in Bond Street, London.

Patients walk in, have the procedure performed under local anaesthetic without the need for any sedation, and walk home 2-3 hours after arrival. We have published our results from the first two years of performing this procedure, showing it is perfectly safe and effective when our protocol is used.

Foam sclerotherapy

Sclerotherapy is the name given to a process where a substance is injected into a vein with a view to destroying it. Sclerotherapy literally comes from Greek "Skleros" meaning "to make hard", and the Latin version of the Greek "Therapia" meaning "a service done to the sick".

For decades, liquid sclerotherapy had been injected into veins with the idea of destroying them. Although successful for very small veins such as thread veins on the legs, this did not work very well in larger veins, particularly those over about 3mm diameter.

The reason for this is because blood destroys the sclerotherapy agent. Sclerotherapy molecules are detergents that work by binding to fat and protein. As cell walls have fat and protein in them, the detergent binds to the cell walls in the walls of the vein, with the aim of destroying the vein itself. Unfortunately, blood is full of cells (red blood cells, white blood cells, platelets) as well as full of fat and protein. Therefore, if blood mixes with sclerotherapy fluid, the sclerotherapy fluid is completely inactivated.

Hence, if liquid sclerotherapy is injected into a big vein, the sclerotherapy merely mixes with the blood causing a clot. This does not damage the vein wall. Once the clot resolves, the vein is still present. Not only does the treatment fail, but the process of getting a clot, followed by clot resolution, often leaves a brown stain on the skin as well! This brown stain is called "haemosiderin".

In 1993, Dr. Juan Cabrera patented a version of sclerotherapy to get around these problems called "microfoam", which is now called foam sclerotherapy. He mixed the sclerosant liquid with air to form a foam, with a consistency a bit like shaving foam. When this is injected into a larger vein, the blood is displaced allowing the sclerotherapy to destroy the vein wall. This seemed to be the answer to treat larger veins.

It soon became clear that injecting air into the veins was not a good idea. Therefore, in good vein clinics, the gas has been changed from air to a combination of carbon dioxide and oxygen, or carbon dioxide alone. These gases are safe to be injected into veins. Published research from The Whiteley Clinic has shown that it is not actually the size of the vein that matters, but the thickness of the vein wall. We have shown that the effects of sclerotherapy can only penetrate about 0.2mm into a vein wall at best.

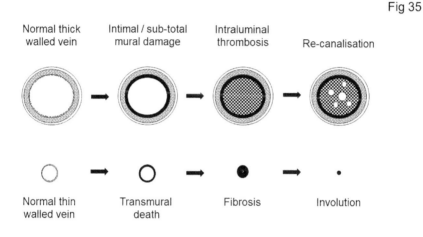

Fig 35

Figure 35: Diagram showing the effects of foam sclerotherapy on the vein wall, in veins with thick walls (top line) and thin walls (lower line). If the vein wall is thick (>0.2mm) then the sclerotherapy only kills the cells on the inner aspect of the vein wall. Blood flowing into the vein will clot. The living cells in the outer part of the vein wall will then work with cells in the blood clot to re-canalise (re-open) the vein. Foam sclerotherapy in veins with thinner walls (<0.2mm) kills all of the cells in the vein wall, leading to fibrosis of the whole vein and disappearance by involution of the whole section of treated vein.

This means that if the vein wall is 0.2mm thick or less, foam sclerotherapy has a chance of working. However, if the vein wall is thicker than this, then only the cells in the inner part of the vein wall will be killed by the foam sclerotherapy, and not the cells further out in the wall. This gives a high chance of a clot forming within the vein, followed by the vein re-opening in the future (Figure 35).

The gonadal veins in the pelvis have wall thicknesses in the region of 0.5mm, as do the internal iliac veins. As such, foam sclerotherapy is not a viable alternative for coil embolisation if these large veins are incompetent.

However, foam sclerotherapy can be used successfully for the treatment of the "stasis veins" and "dilated veins" deep in the pelvis, as these have got thin walls. They can also be used for the veins in the vulva, vagina and perineum which are very tortuous and can only be treated by a foam sclerotherapy approach.

It is for this reason that most patients at The Whiteley Clinic are treated by The Whiteley Protocol which dictates a combination of foam sclerotherapy to the small veins in the bottom of the pelvis, and coil embolisation to the large incompetent veins that are causing the underlying problem.

Glue

Over the last decade or so, there has been an increased use of glue injected into veins to block them permanently. The usual chemical used is cyanoacrylate. Interestingly this is the major chemical used in "superglue". Cyanoacrylate was patented in 1942 but only appeared as an adhesive in 1958. By the 1970s, superglue was being sold to households. As many people found out, it seemed better at sticking fingers together than household objects. In fact, cyanoacrylate glues are much more effective if some moisture is present, as it is in biological tissues.

When injected through catheters into veins, these glues set very quickly (polymerise). If the vein walls can be pushed together, then it will stick the vein together. If not, provided it fills the vein lumen, it will form a permanent plug to permanently ablate the vein. Recent research from The Whiteley Clinic has shown that the superglue completely destroys the inner layer of cells of the vein wall, the endothelium. It is then known that in the long term, the wall of the vein slowly dies away, changing to fibrous tissue. This gives the long-term ablation effects of the glue.

Although many doctors like to use glue, it is less controllable than coils, as these can be seen on x-ray. It is also very expensive. In addition, it really needs the blood to be removed from the vein to get a good adhesion. As such, glue has not become as widespread as coil embolisation for the treatment of pelvic veins.

Plugs

Several companies have developed "plugs" of one sort or another that can be placed within the vein to block it. These range from balloons that can be dilated and then broken off and left in the vein, to different sorts of expandable products that literally plug the vein.

However, as we have discussed previously, our research has shown that venous reflux in both legs and pelvic veins starts at the bottom and works its way upwards. It is an ascending problem. As such, there is no logical place to put a plug. If you plug the top of the vein, this does not treat the origin of the reflux at the bottom.

Additionally, as veins are formed from many tributaries, plugging all of them would require many small plugs. Experience has shown that if a plug is put into a vein at any point, it is likely that a small vein to the side of the main vein will dilate to bypass the plug. Therefore, It is necessary to treat a long length of vein. This can be done with coils, foam and glue. However, for plugs to achieve this, a series of plugs would be needed. This would really get rid of the advantage of using plugs at all.

Other sclerosing agents and gels

There are other sclerosing agents and gels that can be placed deep into the veins in the pelvis, with or without a coil to hold them in place.

Although many have been suggested, few are widely used at the present time. However, as pelvic vein disorder is fast becoming a growth area in phlebology, as more doctors get involved and as more patients realise that they have got curable pelvic congestion syndrome due to pelvic venous disorders, companies will start producing new and more innovative products.

Treatments for pelvic congestion syndrome secondary to venous compression or obstruction

As has been stated several times previously in this book, pelvic congestion syndrome secondary to obstruction or compression appears to be much less common than pelvic reflux disorder.

There are some workers in the field who diagnose compression and obstruction much more commonly then we have found in our long experience. There may be several reasons for this:

- *Patient population* - Different doctors and different practices in different countries have very different patient populations. This can vary from which sort of patients attend the clinic (whether they are predominantly coming with venous problems in the legs and the genitalia, which are found to arise from the pelvis, such as in our clinic; or whether they are predominantly patients with chronic pelvic pain who might be referred from another source for venous investigations), different genetic and familial backgrounds, different medical history with different amounts of previous surgery or venous thrombosis, different body weight and activity level.

- *Investigation method* - As outlined previously, cross-sectional imaging such as MRI/MRV, CT scanning and to an extent venography, are less likely to accurately diagnose venous reflux than duplex ultrasonography, and are more likely to look for compression of veins purely by the look of the vein rather than any functional test.

- *Expertise of the unit or doctor* - Certain doctors become famous for certain techniques and therefore attract referrals from other doctors. These doctors refer because of the expertise of that specialist, and so refer patients most likely to be appropriate for such specialist care. Therefore, if a doctor has become famous for open surgery to bypass compression, and they get referrals from all around the country in patients with that condition, the specialist will start to believe that the compression that they see every day in these referred patients is actually common.

As far as this book is concerned, most patients who are reading it will be suffering from reflux disorder without any compression or obstruction. Most doctors and nurses reading it, unless working in a specialised unit, will also be seeing patients, the majority of which will be suffering from a venous reflux disorder without any compression or obstruction.

Those few patients who are found to have compression will mainly be treatable by opening a vein with a metal tube called a stent. It is only those patients with severe compression or obstruction, who cannot have a stent, that need to go to very specialist centres for open surgery and bypass. Fortunately, this is exceptionally rare.

There has recently been a worrying trend of one or two enthusiasts who believe that compression syndromes are far more common than they are, and who have launched into some very large open surgery operations on patients, with at least one death that is known about from the complications of this open surgery. It is essential that such doctors follow proper medical traditions and publish their results, including their complications. The doctors who are promoting such major surgery without producing evidence are not acting in the best interests of their patients, medical science and in the long term, even themselves.

As venous compressions and obstructions are quite uncommon in patients presenting with pelvic congestion syndrome, and most of those that are found can be treated with stenting, we will now briefly discuss venous stenting. It is beyond the scope of this book to explore the much less common open treatments for compression and obstruction.

Stenting of deep veins

A stent is an expandable metal tube that can be placed within a blood vessel or other tube within the body to hold it open. Many people have heard of "coronary stents" which have been used now for many years to hold coronary arteries open in patients with angina or who have had a heart attack. Stents have been used for a very long time in the artery system.

However, they have only been used more recently in the venous system. As such, most of the current stents were designed to be used in arteries. Hence, there is a lot of research work going on at the moment to optimise stents to be used in veins.

Stents come in two main varieties. Both sorts are placed into position by a long catheter, just the same as the coil catheter for pelvic vein embolisation outlined above. The difference is, rather than a coil being pushed out of the end to block the vein, a stent is deployed to hold a vein open. In some cases, if the vein is completely blocked, or if the vein is very narrow, a balloon is put in first to open or dilate the vein before the stent is placed.

The two different sorts of stents are those that have to be expanded when they are being placed, and those that are self-expanding. The first sort tends to be put on a balloon and when the balloon is dilated, the stent is also stretched and positioned in the vein, pushing outwards on the vein wall. The second, the self-expanding stent, is usually made of a memory metal (nitinol) and is squashed into a very small tube and placed into the catheter. When it is pushed out of the end of the catheter, it self-expands into place pushing open the vein.

An example of how a stent might be used in an iliac occlusion such as that pictured in Figure 27, is shown in Figure 36.

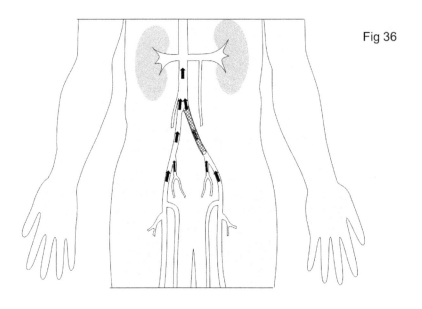

Fig 36

Figure 36: Diagram showing how a stent might be used to open an occluded vein such as that illustrated in the previous Figure 27.

When a vein is completely blocked or very narrowed, with obvious obstructive symptoms and signs (2AO), then a stent is a very good option if the patient is suitable and accepting. However, in the surgical world at the present time, there is a concern about putting stents into young people who have many years ahead of them, for compressions that might only be mild or insignificant. In these cases, the stent can interact with the vein wall over many years causing the vein wall to thicken and narrow or even block.

Now that we have explored treatments, we have enough knowledge to start putting things together in the final chapter. We will start to think about how patients should be investigated, and which patients should be treated and by what techniques.

Chapter 8

What Treatments, for Which Patients and What Outcomes?

Pelvic congestion syndrome (PCS), particularly when proven to be from pelvic venous disorders (PVeD), is still a very new area of study in the medical world. If you have followed all of the arguments to this point in the book, you will have as much knowledge as most people who are involved in pelvic congestion syndrome work, and indeed much more than most doctors and nurses who have undergone normal medical and nursing training. This is because there is almost nothing taught about this condition to students nor junior doctors and nurses.

Further evidence that this is so new, is shown by the fact that when I started this book, I typed "pelvic congestion syndrome" into Amazon - and found virtually nothing at all! No books with "pelvic congestion syndrome" in the title were offered at all! My own book "Advances in Phlebology and Venous Surgery Volume 1" that has two chapters on pelvic congestion syndrome due to pelvic venous disorders, was one of the few that were offered. Most of the other books were more related to musculoskeletal pelvic pain than anything to do with pelvic congestion syndrome and pelvic venous disorders.

The good thing about new specialities like this is that we are able to diagnose people who have not been given diagnoses previously, and are able to offer treatments to those who thought, or who had been told, that they were incurable (or in some cases that there was nothing wrong with them!).

However, the bad thing about new specialities like this is that because it is new and research is actively going forwards, we don't know everything about the condition yet. Hence when we discuss treatments with patients, we often have to explain that we are playing the odds, and nothing is certain. This is why informed consent is so very important, and why patients need to make 100% sure they are happy with the doctors who are treating them, and the techniques that they are being offered, for both investigation and treatment.

So, let us look at different presentations of pelvic congestion syndrome, what investigations should be offered, what treatments should be offered and what results should be expected.

The primary problem - Pelvic congestion symptoms (1A and/or 1B)

Patients presenting with the symptoms of pelvic congestion syndrome as their primary concern, whether inside the pelvis (1A) and/or outside of the pelvis (1B), fall into three main groups (Figure 37). There is also a fourth group that we need to think about. In this fourth group, the patients do not have any 1A or 1B symptoms, but they do have proven pelvic venous reflux. The reason we must consider these patients will become clear below.

The first group is patients who have symptoms that could be due to pelvic congestion syndrome (1A and/or 1B). When the transvaginal duplex ultrasound scan is performed using the Holdstock-Harrison protocol, no significant pelvic reflux is found, and no pelvic varicose veins are identified. Compression can be checked for using transabdominal duplex and the Holdstock-White protocol, but if there is no reflux and no dilated veins in the pelvis, it is likely that there is no pelvic venous disorder present.

Therefore, although these patients present with the symptoms of pelvic congestion syndrome, they do not have pelvic venous disorder and other causes for their symptoms must be looked for by relevant specialists depending on the symptom profile.

Jumping to the last group (Figure 37), there are patients who do not complain of any symptoms of pelvic congestion syndrome (1A or 1B), but are incidentally found to have pelvic venous reflux when they are being investigated for other conditions, most commonly leg varicose veins (2B) or varicose veins of the vulva and vagina (2A). The reason it is important to think about these patients is that this group proves that there are patients who have significant pelvic venous reflux but who do not have pelvic symptoms (1A or 1B). Once we have understood this, we can then make sense of the advice we give patients in the second group, which we are now about to discuss.

Fig 37

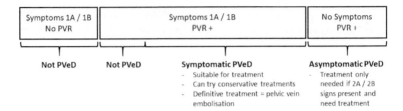

Figure 37: A simple way of thinking about how patients with Pelvic Congestion Syndrome (PCS) and/or Pelvic Venous Disorders (PVeD) might present. It highlights that symptoms and venous disorders are not always linked. This is particularly important in patients who have symptoms (1A, 1B) and are found to have a pelvic venous disorder (PVeD) but, the PVeD is only incidental and so treatment does not cure the symptoms (see text).

So, turning to the second group, this is the group of patients who have the symptoms suggestive of pelvic congestion syndrome (1A and/or 1B), who are then proven to have significant pelvic vein reflux on transvaginal venous duplex ultrasonography using the Holdstock-Harrison protocol. It would appear at first glance that these patients have symptomatic pelvic congestion syndrome due to their proven pelvic venous disorder, which in this case is pelvic venous reflux. As such it is pretty obvious that treatment of this reflux should cure the patient.

Although this is true for the majority of these patients, there is a sub-group within this group in which it is not the case. We have already seen that in the first group some patients can have symptoms that suggest pelvic congestion syndrome but turn out not to have any pelvic venous abnormality. In the last group, we can also see that some patients have significant pelvic venous reflux but do not have any pelvic symptoms.

Therefore, it is not surprising that some patients who present with the symptoms of pelvic congestion syndrome, and who have proven pelvic venous reflux, might actually have their pelvic symptoms for other reasons and the pelvic venous reflux is actually incidental and not related to the symptoms at all.

It is this sub-group that means that whilst we assess patients by their symptoms and then look for pelvic venous reflux, we will never get 100% cure rate until we can find a test that can positively link any pelvic vein reflux that is identified, to the exact symptoms it is causing.

Therefore, when these patients are consented for pelvic vein embolisation, it is essential that they understand that even if the embolisation is technically perfect, it is possible that some or all of the symptoms might remain. These symptoms are the ones that were not due to the venous disorder in the first place.

As such, any patient undergoing pelvic vein embolisation who has any residual symptoms, needs to have a post embolisation transvaginal venous duplex ultrasound scan performed using the Holdstock-Harrison protocol, 4-8 weeks after the pelvic vein embolisation. This test will tell whether the remaining symptoms are due to a technical failure of the embolisation (such as the coils being left too high in the vein, insufficient coils being placed along the vein or the incorrect veins being embolised) or whether they are not due to venous causes.

Finally in this section, and as noted previously in this book, it is surprising how many patients undergo pelvic vein embolisation for signs alone (either leg varicose veins – 2B - or external varicose veins around the pelvis – 2A) without any pelvic symptoms, who then tell us post-embolisation that their pelvic symptoms have massively improved. As noted previously, when patients live with chronic discomfort for a very long time, sometimes it becomes accepted as normal and relief is only noticed when the discomfort is removed.

Patients presenting with varicose veins around the genitalia, perineum, buttocks, anus, lower abdomen or flanks (2A)

Of all of the patient groups, this is the most diverse.

As we have previously discussed, patients who have prominent varicose veins across the pubic area or lower abdomen, or ascending up the flanks from the pelvis towards the chest, are classically due to obstructed deep veins in the pelvis and abdomen. These signs are almost universally due to obstruction of the main veins, and hence these patients can be termed 2AO - where the O is for obstruction.

These patients should go straight to doctors who are interested in stenting or operating on the deep veins. Most of these patients have a long history of previous deep vein thromboses (DVT's) or who have had other major interventions such as abdominal or pelvic surgery, radiotherapy, interventions into the veins in the groin and so forth. This is a special group of patients that usually know there is something going on in their deep venous system and very rarely present to doctors as a possible pelvic congestion syndrome patient.

Patients who have haemorrhoids tend to go directly to colorectal surgeons, or coloproctologists. At the present time, there are several treatments for haemorrhoids that are minimally invasive and that generally ablate the haemorrhoid veins and surrounding tissue with heat (radiofrequency or laser being the most common), or the veins alone with sclerotherapy or foam sclerotherapy techniques. Research in the future will tell whether these veins would be better treated by checking for pelvic venous reflux as well. However, at the current time, if haemorrhoids are the only problem the patient has, this is probably the right way they should be treated.

Males who have varicoceles have traditionally presented to urologists because they deal with the testicles and external genitalia of the male. The traditional treatment is open surgery to tie (ligate) the testicular vein. Fortunately, increasing numbers of these patients are now being referred to interventional radiologists who work in venous centres, so the testicular veins can be embolised using the principles discussed in the last chapter.

Females who have varicose veins of their perineum, buttocks or external genitalia (including labia, vulva and vagina), need to undergo transvaginal venous duplex ultrasound scanning using the Holdstock-Harrison protocol. Any reflux found will require the extended transabdominal dupex scan using the Holdstock-White Protocol, to look for the uncommon compression or obstruction syndromes. Treatment will then be determined as to which of the four major veins are refluxing, or if the varicose veins are localised and not been fed by major pelvic vein reflux.

As noted before, erectile dysfunction in men may also soon fall into this group. It is still very early days for this and so, for this edition of the book, we will leave erectile dysfunction alone at present.

Patients presenting with leg varicose veins found to be arising from pelvic venous reflux (2B)

These are the patients that we have most experience with, having been treating them now for 20 years. It is well recognised that approximately 20% of women with leg varicose veins have a contribution from pelvic varicose veins, with 16.7% having pelvic vein reflux as the underlying cause. In men, we have recently published that this also affects 3% of men presenting with leg varicose veins.

Although no randomised study has so far been performed, we have published our own research showing that one of the most common causes of recurrent varicose veins after varicose veins surgery, is untreated pelvic vein reflux at the initial operation. Other research groups who have started looking into this using adequate methodology are finding the same results.

Therefore, to get the best results for patients who have leg varicose veins that require treatment, a venous duplex ultrasound of the leg should always include an assessment as to whether venous reflux is entering the leg from the pelvis. In patients where this is found to be the case, they should be offered a transvaginal venous duplex ultrasound scan using the Holdstock-Harrison protocol.

If this shows significant pelvic vein reflux, then all the current evidence would suggest that pelvic vein embolisation should be offered to reduce the risk of recurrent varicose veins in the future. If the patient has incidental external pelvic varicose veins classic of pelvic vein reflux (2AR) such as varicose veins of the vulva, vagina or labia, or indeed any symptoms suggestive of pelvic congestion syndrome (1A and/or 1B) these may well improve as a side effect of this treatment. This would be a bonus but not the primary reason to offer pelvic vein embolisation in these cases.

Over the last few years, we have had several patients through The Whiteley Clinic who have presented with varicose veins or recurrent varicose veins of the legs, and who have been found to have pelvic venous reflux as a major cause of their leg varicose veins, but who have then refused to have pelvic vein embolisation. This is contrary to The Whiteley Protocol, where Stage I treatment aims to ablate all abnormal venous reflux. However, patient consent is paramount and so these patients are warned that in our view, they have a higher risk of recurrent varicose veins of the legs in the future. Provided they accept this we then proceed to treat them as they request.

Our experience is that most start finding recurrent varicose veins in the legs arising from the pelvis after 1-3 years.

When presenting at international meetings, some doctors suggest that in patients with leg varicose veins associated with proven pelvic vein reflux, it might be best to treat the leg varicose veins first. They then suggest that they will only go on to treat the pelvic vein reflux if the patient subsequently gets recurrent varicose veins.

Indeed, this idea was recently put forward by Dr Rosenblatt in a commentary on our research paper about men with leg varicose veins with associated pelvic vein reflux, in the journal "Phlebology". As we answered him in a letter to the editor, and as I reply to such comments at international meetings, although this sounds good to doctors, most patients don't agree when they realise what it means to them. It means that patients undergo leg varicose vein treatments first, and then when the leg varicose veins recur, they not only have to undergo pelvic vein embolisation, but also have to have their leg varicose veins treated a second time!

Of course, if the patient accepts this as a likely result of the initial strategy, then that is not a problem. They need to be happy to consent to that process, including accepting the time, cost and risks of a second varicose veins procedure. My personal preference is to give the best treatment first time around, with the lowest possible risk of recurrence in the future. However, until randomised controlled studies have been performed (assuming that they ever will be) patients must be informed of both possible routes forward and must consent to the pros and cons of whichever route they take.

Having gone through that in some detail, of course most doctors who treat varicose veins do not even check for pelvic vein reflux in their patients. Therefore, they do not offer pelvic vein embolisation to their patients as neither doctor nor patient knows about the presence of the pelvic vein reflux. As such, the patients never have to worry about whether to consent for the embolisation or not, but conversely it is one of the major reasons that patients still have high recurrence rates after varicose vein surgery!

Long-term results and effects on fertility

At The Whiteley Clinic we have now been performing pelvic vein embolisation for 20 years. Although 20 years is a long time to humans, as far as medicine is concerned it is quite a brief history for a condition. Although our research has answered a great many questions, the fact that very few doctors are looking into this problem, never mind treating it, means that there is not a huge amount of data coming through to tease out some of the nuances of the condition.

Two of the common questions that are frequently asked, are about the long-term effects of the coils, and the effects on fertility of having coil embolisation of the ovarian veins.

With regards to the long-term results, we have published a series of patients that we followed up eight years after their embolisation. We showed an excellent closure of the treated veins with some new pelvic vein reflux developing in veins that had previously been normal. The levels that we found this in are in keeping with what we would expect as the natural deterioration in people who are prone to develop varicose veins. There was no evidence of any detrimental effect in the long term from having the coils in the body.

With regards to fertility, many women are concerned that embolising the ovarian vein might affect ovarian function. In fact, it only takes a minute to think about the physiology to realise that this is exactly the wrong way around. The ovaries take their blood supply from the ovarian arteries, and these are not affected by pelvic vein embolisation.

However, what actually happens is different. The venous blood is not being taken away from the ovaries, but instead, due to the reflux in the incompetent ovarian vein, the venous blood is remaining in dilated veins around the ovary. Surrounding the ovary with venous stasis can only be detrimental to the ovarian function.

Therefore, pelvic vein embolisation in patients with severe pelvic venous reflux and ovarian varicoceles is likely to improve ovarian function. Moreover, as pain during sexual intercourse (deep dyspareunia) is one of the internal pelvic symptoms of pelvic congestion syndrome due to pelvic venous disorders (1A), treatment of the pelvic veins and resolution of this pain is likely to improve the chances of getting pregnant.

Conclusions and Last Thoughts

It is very frustrating for patients suffering from chronic pelvic pain and the other symptoms and signs of pelvic congestion syndrome, that there are so few doctors who specialise in venous diseases and who are interested in finding out more about this common condition.

As I have already written in this book, this means that worldwide, millions of women are either being ignored or are getting the wrong advice and treatments. Increasingly, we are finding this is probably true for men too.

We have pretty good data to show that between 13-40% of women attending gynaecology clinics with chronic pelvic pain have pelvic congestion syndrome (PCS) due to pelvic venous disorder (PVeD). This means that they could be cured if they had the right investigations and treatment. Instead these patients often get diagnosed with endometriosis or get told that there is nothing wrong with them.

Because most doctors who treat leg varicose veins do not look for nor treat pelvic vein reflux, 1 in 6 women and 1 in 30 men get inadequate assessment and treatment of leg varicose veins, leading to a much higher chance of recurrence.

Improvements in the understanding of pelvic venous disorders and possible new investigations and treatments, increases the chances of improved treatments for haemorrhoids, with a low recurrence rate in the future. There is also the possibility of the treatment of some forms of erectile dysfunction, just around the corner.

Overall, even with the knowledge we have at the moment, millions of people are not getting the relief of symptoms and signs of pelvic congestion syndrome because the knowledge in this book is not being widely disseminated into the medical community, and most doctors are generalists and do not go to specialist conferences.

A recent publication from England by Prof Bruce Campbell has shown how poorly this is understood by vascular surgeons. He and his colleagues showed that a proportion of doctors who treat leg varicose veins either do not believe pelvic venous reflux has any effect on leg varicose veins or, if they do believe it, do not do anything to investigate or treat it. Even in those who do treat it, the vast majority treat fewer than 10 cases a year. In no other area of medicine would this be deemed an acceptable number to keep up sufficient experience to do a good job.

At international conferences, lectures are still given by invited "experts" who still come out with information and statements that are clearly incorrect. The most common is that pelvic congestion syndrome is a condition found in women who have had children! At every opportunity I stand up and ask the "expert" how they explain that men get varicoceles, as far as I am aware, very few men have children! This is easier than pointing out all the hundreds of women we have successfully treated who have never had children.

The problem when there is any gap in authoritative medical knowledge is that many people with different agendas, but no actual research data tend to try to influence thought processes.

With the advent of social media, this is a major problem as it is so easy to set up a group on the Internet and post opinion as if it is fact. If patients suffering from the condition in question are not getting good medical advice, they will accept this opinion as if it were fact, particularly if the posts are regular and worded strongly.

I have every sympathy with the well-meaning patients who partake in these activities because they have either had very poor experiences themselves, in getting doctors to listen to them or treat them.

However, in amongst these well-meaning people, there are many others with different agendas who the public need to be very wary of.

Some are obvious, such as those offering "miracle cures" that can be purchased over the Internet such as herbal remedies, tablets or teas. Hopefully having read this book, you will be well aware that none of these will affect venous reflux nor the rarer venous compression in any meaningful way.

Others are more concerning. I am particularly concerned at the moment by reports of open surgery for multiple "compressions" of the pelvic and abdominal veins, giving miraculous cures. There is even a lecture by a doctor that was given at an international meeting, that was posted on the internet.

However, no data can be found in respected peer-reviewed journals for this approach and, at the time of going to press with this book, there are no peer-reviewed results and no complications quoted. I am aware of at least one patient who died having had this sort of open surgery, and yet this patient does not appear in any presentation that I have seen so far.

Therefore, any person who has the symptoms or signs of pelvic congestion syndrome needs to obtain as much information as they can about their condition, and then assess all sources for credibility. Any proper scientific source should be able to back up their arguments with their own research papers, published in peer-reviewed journals.

As far as doctors are concerned, it is clear that the current position where most doctors do not understand or know about pelvic congestion should be changed, and this should be taught as part of training schemes. Those of us who are engaged in the assessment and treatment of patients should all be trained on recognised training courses such as those we have set up at The Whiteley Clinic and through the College of Phlebology.

Doctors who investigate and treat patients with pelvic congestion syndrome from pelvic venous disorders should work in groups where results are kept, analysed and published. Any complications or adverse outcomes must be discussed, and lessons learnt. As with all medical conditions, doctors performing fewer than 10 cases per year should either join units where they can increase their experience or should refer patients to units that perform higher numbers and who have support, back up and experience.

We have set up the International Venous Registry through the College of Phlebology. This allows any doctor who is treating patients with pelvic venous disorders to submit their own figures, in order that their practice and results can be benchmarked against other doctors in the world who treat the same sort of patients. This registry includes all of the information about the treatment, the doctor's assessment of outcome and, most importantly, the patient's reported outcome.

The registry e-mails patients regularly to check that they have had a good result but, unlike many satisfaction type websites, it continues to do so over the years to check what the recurrence rates are from different doctors and different techniques. Patients would be well advised to look for the College of Phlebology Venous Registry Logo on any doctor's website, or just log onto the College of Phlebology website (www.collegeofphlebology.com) where all doctors who are actively involved in the registry are listed.

Continuing research into pelvic congestion syndrome and pelvic venous disorders, along with registry data, will result in patients getting better diagnoses and results in the long term.

I hope that this book has been useful to you, whether you are a patient or a healthcare professional, and it stimulates you to get more interested in this fascinating area.

If you are a patient, it will help you identify the best route forward for your investigations and treatments and will help you know if you are getting optimal care. It will arm you with the knowledge to ask pertinent questions if you believe that you are not.

If you are a healthcare professional, it should help you understand what the optimal investigations and treatments are currently, and give you a framework of the rationale as to why we treat pelvic congestion syndrome the way we do at the current time.

I am very happy to be contacted and provide a list of references to any interested parties.

Mark Whiteley, September 2019

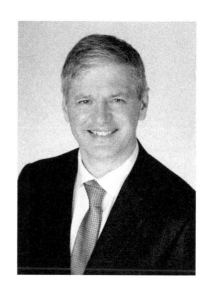

About the Author

Prof Mark S Whiteley is an internationally recognised expert in venous diseases including pelvic congestion syndrome related to pelvic venous disorders. He is one of the authors on the recent International Consensus Document on Pelvic Congestion Syndrome from the UIP.

Mark performed the first endovenous surgery for varicose veins in the UK in March 1999 and started researching pelvic venous disorders in 2000. He set up The Whiteley Clinic as a centre of excellence in venous disorders in 2002 and The College of Phlebology to share his knowledge with patients and other health care professionals in 2011.

In 2019 he set up The College of Phlebology International Registry so that doctors who join can benchmark their results against other doctors doing the same procedures, and patients can see which medical professionals are getting acceptable results from their treatments.

Mark continues to work to bring new ideas and technology to venous patients, to improve results and get the best outcomes possible.

CPSIA information can be obtained
at www.ICGtesting.com
Printed in the USA
BVHW040859151019
561140BV00015B/290/P